abortion
counseling
and
social change

abortion counseling and social change

from illegal act to medical practice

THE STORY OF THE
CLERGY CONSULTATION SERVICE
ON ABORTION

ARLENE CARMEN
and HOWARD MOODY

Judson Press, Valley Forge

ABORTION COUNSELING AND SOCIAL CHANGE

Copyright © 1973
Judson Press, Valley Forge, Pa. 19481

Library of Congress Cataloging in Publication Data

Carmen, Arlene.
    Abortion counseling and social change.
        1. Abortion—United States. 2. Pastoral counseling.
I. Moody, Howard, joint author. II. Title.
[DNLM: 1. Abortion, Induced. 2. Counseling.
3. Social change. HQ 767 C287a 1973]
HQ767.5.U5C37   261.8   72-11221
ISBN O-8170-0579-X

Printed in the U.S.A.

DEDICATED TO

The congregation of Judson Church
without whose encouragement and
forbearance this odyssey would
have been impossible

Preface

There is a great deal of difference between living *in* history and recalling history. We are attempting to set down here a living record of the birth and development of an organization not for itself but for what it might teach us of our attitudes, the changing of institutions, and the reform of laws.

The sources of information for this record are simply some documents and our memories. Those who believe that the memory operates on the model of a camera with an objective lens registering each event in one's past will be sorely disappointed in what must be a faulty "machine." But those who know, as we do, that the memory is far from being an accurate historical recorder but is, rather, a censor and editor of the past, selecting events which *our* biases and prejudices covet, will understand the gaps and omissions in this chronicle. Events, causative factors, and people's names are missing not because they were unimportant but because our view of what happened in the process was not total but partial and distorted. Others may have a different perspective and might want to tell the story in a different fashion.

Our hope is that this chronicle and its interpretation may enable others, as it enabled us, to see the complexity of change, how change happens sometimes *because* of its champions but more often *in spite* of them. This is not just a book about *abortion,* but it is about people, their laws, their prejudices, and what sometimes changes them.

ARLENE CARMEN
HOWARD MOODY

Acknowledgments

We would like especially to pay tribute to the enormous contribution of all the clergy and lay persons who for the past five years have given time and concern to women with unwanted pregnancies. Our special thanks to Joan Muyskens, secretary of Judson Church, who many times shared our work far beyond the call of duty; and to Mrs. Harvey McClintock, whose generosity and encouragement enabled the National Clergy Consultation Service to grow and expand its services.

Contents

The Dark Ages: Man's Vengeance on Woman — The Penalty for an Unwanted Pregnancy

We now find it hard to realize that only a short time ago the word "abortion" was not used in normal conversation. Those who had experienced abortions knew and belonged to a large sodality of women which had no secret handshakes or symbols and whose members only accidentally knew each other. But members of this group were more numerous than those attracted to the ranks of the later women's liberation movement. Somewhere in the personal history of millions of women in this nation there was an ugly, traumatic drama stashed in the bank of unforgettable memories. It was an *illicit abortion.*

Even though the dark ages of pre-abortion reform was only a few years ago, we will need to put ourselves back into that time to recall what it was like for a woman to have an unwanted pregnancy and desire to terminate it. What happened to her at that time? Even in a state with a law as strict as New York, a woman who had "connections" (a doctor friend, a psychiatrist) and *money* could, in a New York hospital, terminate the pregnancy under the guise of a "therapeutic abortion." It is important to understand the terminology that medical and legal persons invented to rationalize the ignoring of the law in certain cases. The term "therapeutic" was both hypocritical and euphemistic. It was used to describe an abortion that was ascertained as necessary to "save the life of the mother," that being the only legal reason for the act. "Therapeutic," as used by the medical profession, was a term of justification. In fact it was only a term to describe the difference between rich and poor, white and black, the privileged and the underprivileged, married and single.

Almost all of the abortions performed under this rubric could not by any stretch of the imagination or language be construed to fall under legal justification. In 1967 in most of the states a "therapeutic abortion" simply meant a "legal" abortion in contrast to a so-called "criminal" abortion. This phony distinction and widespread practice of discriminatory abortions was one of the impelling reasons which led us not only to fight for the reform of the law but also to consider seriously the "disobedience" of the law. Not only were "legal" therapeutic abortions done in hospitals, but "illegal" abortions were also performed there, i.e., abortions done without formal acknowledgment of hospital personnel. Several large hospitals had "under the table" arrangements to do first trimester (within the first twelve weeks of pregnancy) abortions which cost somewhere between $1,500 and $2,000. The desperation of women was enough to encourage a black market even in "therapeutic abortions." These were a kind of "illegal" legal abortion. If you understand these fine distinctions, you could have been a legislator in New York State in 1967.

But what about those women without means, unmarried, very young, or poor, or black? How did they get abortions? They relied on the "grapevine." The "grapevine" is the interconnected, survival cord in the illicit underground which develops to fulfill any prohibited need. In this case, it was a list of "abortionists," passed from hand to hand, usually on college campuses or among single women in large metropolitan areas. In those days, an individual clergyman who had experience in counseling women in difficulty (and there were practically no such clergy) had the names of several "doctors" who for $500 or $600 would perform an abortion. A major disadvantage and even danger of the list was that each person who referred women sent so few that there was no effective method of checking on these "abortionists" and the medical procedure they were using. The known list of persons performing abortions was long. There were, of course, the celebrities like Dr. Spencer in Pennsylvania, Dr. Rappaport in New York, and Dr. Raymond in New Jersey, but unfortunately for women the medical credentials and experience of the lesser known "doctors" were not verifiable. Those women, mostly poor and members of minority groups, who had no access to the grapevine had their own prescriptions for self-induced abortions, which often resulted in sterilization and death; or they used the services of a practicing midwife who lived in the ghetto.

If we look at the experience of those women who were "lucky" enough to have access to the grapevine, we may be able to understand the psychic scars that probably contributed to the psychiatric profession's "mythology" regarding the ill effects on the mental health of women who had abortions. The fear and shame of the criminalizing process, having to do something that was made to appear "dirty" and "unsavory" in order to achieve some control of her life, the physical pain that came from what was often the absence of anaesthesia, the anxiety that came from not knowing the credentials or the skills of the practitioner—all of these factors increased immeasurably the psychic pain and physical suffering of a woman forced to resort to this kind of solution by a medical/legal system that simply did not care.

Let's look at a typical situation in New York of a woman who took the route of illegal abortion in the time before abortion reform or professional counseling and referral were available. The woman called a phone number, and a man answered. He said he was busy, but he would call back if she would leave her number. This man was not a doctor but a "middleman" in the abortion business who worked for the "doctor" and was paid a set amount for each woman he referred to the "doctor." He called her back and told her how much money she needed to bring in cash and made arrangements to pick her up somewhere in Manhattan. When they met, he took her to an office where the procedure was performed. The woman never knew in advance where she was to be taken nor did she know the name or the qualifications of the person performing the procedure. Like most women in this situation, she was *not* permitted to bring a relative or friend along with her. Her anxiety was thus compounded by the anxiety of those closest to her who, had she not returned, would have had no information about where she was or whom she was with. Since both the name and the phone number of the "middleman" were constantly changing, his whereabouts would have been hard to trace.

This situation, believe it or not, was one of the better ones. Other women wound up in motel rooms where a so-called doctor would do the procedure on the bed while the woman was blindfolded so as not to discover his identity. He would do the procedure and disappear. The woman, still blindfolded, would be driven back to the parking lot where she was picked up; the whole transaction would take place in complete silence except for the cries of pain and shame from the lips of the victim. If she was very fortunate, had lots of money but no hospital connections, she might have her abortion done in a luxurious hotel suite by a Park Avenue doctor, using an alias, with nurses in attendance. The cost would be about $1,000 for such an abortion. Some loss of dignity might be spared the woman in this kind of situation, but her anxiety was probably no less. It is hard to imagine an experience more traumatizing or dehumanizing for a woman or more likely to have a deleterious effect on her psychic health.

One of the most sophisticated and humane abortion rings we encountered in those days operated out of Washington, D.C. It consisted of a group of very reputable doctors in the Washington/Baltimore area. The "middleman" was a charming, middle-aged Southerner by whom we were contacted. In this procedure the pregnant woman was picked up at the train or plane by a limousine driven by the "middleman." The limousine had a two-way radio that enabled him to keep in constant touch with the doctors and receive calls from the patients as they arrived in the city. When a woman was picked up, she paid the money to the "middleman" in the car. He then transferred her money to a brown envelope addressed to the "accountant" for the business and dropped it in a mailbox. (This way the doctors never touched the patient's money.) At the end of each week the "accountant" wrote checks for all the staff including the "middleman," who was paid a flat fee for every patient he delivered to the doctors. A number of women who went through this procedure were recruited to be agents in their town or on their campus. As agents they would receive a "kickback" of $25-$50 for each woman they sent to the Washington doctors. In this way the ring was able to establish a network which seemed to operate throughout the southern part of the United States. The existence of this network explained why, at least in the experience of the clergy, women in the South seemed able to attain abortions without a professional counseling service. We suspected, but never knew, that the ring had some connections or understandings with Washington authorities since it operated in a relatively open and public way.

One of the interesting phenomena of the illicit abortion business in the United States was that the "Mafia" or the underworld syndicate never moved into the field and dominated it even though it was a multimillion dollar business annually. It may be a little cynical to suggest that the reason the "Mafia" stayed out was on moral and religious grounds, but it is hard to find another explanation. The only place that seemed an exception to this rule was the state of New Jersey where there was evidence of outside controls over doctors and "middlemen."

In these dark days of pre-abortion reform one might ask where the medical profession was in a matter almost completely medical by nature. That profession was paralyzed by prejudice (against abortion as life-negating), fear (of losing their licenses), and ignorance (most of them had only delivered babies). When a patient discovered that she was accidentally pregnant, even when the obstetrician-gynecologist was her personal doctor and had prescribed the contraceptives, the physician became nonfunctional as far as that patient was concerned. Often a doctor refused to discuss the "problem," pretending the patient was a stranger; he would not suggest alternatives but would merely suggest that if she planned to go through with the foolish notion of having an abortion she could "come back and see me when it is all over." We met many an angry and disillusioned woman in those days who had believed that her physician really cared about her only to discover at the moment of this terrible medical and ethical dilemma that he offered neither medical help nor even moral support.

The attitude of doctors toward those persons in the profession who became "abortionists" was one of absolute contempt. This attitude was held even by those doctors who were "liberal" enough to refer wealthy patients to them. One of the great failures of those in the medical profession who did refer women to or give them phone numbers of "abortionists" is that, because of their desire to be medically pure, they refused to "police" or call into account, in any way, the colleagues whom they considered pariahs of the profession unfit for licensing but whom they used to perform a medical service which they refused their patients. The hypocrisy and double standards of many in the medical profession were exceeded only by their irresponsibility toward their women patients whose health and life depended on these "abortionists."

In all fairness it must be said that probably a majority of the profession in those days did not believe that abortion was right for everyone; they did not refer women because they did not believe that women should have abortions except for the most compelling reasons. Abortion certainly was not a medical procedure that most doctors felt a woman was entitled to by request. It was the conservatism of the medical profession as much as that of the legislators that kept the harsh, restrictive laws on the books until the latter part of the twentieth century.

A word should be said here about the "illegal abortionist" whose *genre* was generated by the law of supply and demand that accompanies every prohibitionistic culture that makes certain personal services and needs "illegal" and "criminal." It should be noted here that nomenclature is very revealing. The "abortionist," as the doctor was called, was a term of opprobrium approved by the medical profession for putting him outside the pale. But when the law changed and abortions were legal, a physician who worked full time in an abortion clinic was never called an "abortionist" even though he performed the same services.

These doctors who were performing at that time outside of accepted medical practice and procedures were cut off from their profession in every way. All the checks and balances that come from medical practice in the acceptable forms had to be missing while at the same time these doctors were earning more money than their colleagues. All of this produced a certain pathology contributed to by the illegal nature of the practice as well as being "dumped on" by their profession. Many of them deserved the unsavory reputation they earned, but we found later that not all of them were as bad as their "reputation." It does seem unfair that the psychiatric profession gave a great deal of study and attention to the "personality disorders" and psychological problems of women who had unwanted pregnancies or abortions, but on the other hand never studied the problems or pathology of medical men engaged in a lucrative business that thrived on the desperation and misery of helpless women.

We heard countless lectures in those days about how damaging to one's mental health abortion really was. Many psychiatrists, buttressed by studies and the reports of other doctors, prolonged that myth without reference to the social context in which the abortion actually occurred. It was similar to another myth about women which the psychiatric profession encouraged and that was about "unwanted pregnancies" which were really "wanted" in order to hurt somebody or punish someone. Many psychiatrists believed devoutly that all so-called unwanted pregnancies were forms of acting out anti-socially or rebelling against parents. Very few were willing to admit that the reasons a woman became pregnant when she preferred not to be had to do with a whole complex of problems related to unsatisfactory sex education, inadequate birth control measures, the heavy moral burden placed on single women if they performed sexually out of marriage, and most importantly related to a way in which men looked at women and put them in their place.

When one looks back even over the space of a few years and sees what women were put through in order to pay lip service to a discriminatory and outmoded statute, one can only conclude that abortion was directly calculated, whether consciously or not, to be an excessive, cruel, and unnecessary punishment, physically and psychologically, of women.

In 1967 Al Blumenthal, the Chairman of the Health Codes Committee of the New York State Assembly, was trying to get out of his Committee onto the floor of the legislature a mild abortion reform bill. Early that year a small group of clergy, under the impetus and encouragement of Lawrence Lader, a longtime proponent of abortion law change, had conversations about what we would do to help women if the legislature failed to act. The suggestion put forth was to establish a counseling service to assist women in the difficult time of an unwanted pregnancy. The final blow, giving impetus to the clergy, was the refusal of the lawmakers even to let the bill out of committee. It seemed to us ironical that the legislators who refused even to talk about reforming the law were all men who had never been pregnant, and the group of persons preparing to give aid and counsel to the women were clergy (mostly men) who belonged to an institution that was more responsible than most for the law staying on the books.

Those of us clergy in New York City who had gathered together at the Washington Square Methodist Church in the early spring of 1967 did so out of some strong convictions that leadership for the reform of that heartless and inequitable law should come from those of us who preached justice without demanding it and admonished mercy without giving it. It seemed to us only right that the counseling, encouragement, and assistance which women needed under this unjust law should come from that institution, the Christian church, so responsible for the origins and perpetuation of that law.

Consciousness Raising with the Clergy

Lawrence Lader, who had already written his earliest book, *Abortion,* was the first to suggest that it would perhaps be a significant gesture if the clergy were to refer women directly to places where they might obtain abortions, such as he had been doing by telephone and letter for some time. Out of Lader's encouragement was born the first concept of what later would become the Clergy Consultation Service on Abortion. Discussions of what we might be willing to do led us to call together a group of clergy to whom we would present the idea of developing a counseling and referral service while at the same time educating ourselves as to what might be done eventually regarding the law.

It was apparent from the start that the clergy who would be most likely to become involved in a project of this kind would be the same ones who had been most active in the school integration battle in New York, in the civil rights battle both there and in the South, as well as in other areas of civil liberties. It was to those clergy whose liberal attitudes and commitments had been clearly established that we turned for help in developing the original nucleus of the Clergy Consultation Service on Abortion. We invited about forty people to our first meeting, and about twenty or twenty-five persons attended. It was obvious from that initial get-together that, though some felt a keen interest, many felt that abortion was a problem about which they knew very little, and hardly any felt pressure from their congregations or communities to make this issue a priority. This attitude was reminiscent of the early days of the civil rights movement when people would say they didn't have a Negro problem in *their* community because there weren't any Negroes. The reaction of this group of clergy to the abortion issue stemmed from a poor understanding and limited knowledge of the problem as well as a failure to realize that if they were to make themselves available to women experiencing this problem they would discover needs they never knew existed. Clearly our first order of business had to be *self-education*. We could not enjoy the luxury of moving into this unknown territory of emotional and psychological strain without a depth of investigation which had to include the opening of our minds to experiences we had never known. Clergymen are predisposed by training and intellect to deal in answers and categories with which they have background and experience, theological and pastoral ethics. Here was a field in which ministers and rabbis had very little experience. And those clergy who did have some experience in this field, because of both religious and cultural prejudices, usually counseled against a woman opting for an abortion. Later, most of us were to see theological "principles" and ethical norms shattered by the existential burden of a decision that cried not for sermons and exhortations but for supportive affirmation and concrete assistance for the person.

Almost all projects of service which are aimed at a constituency that one wants to help demand a process of immersion in the "problem" before one decides what form an action must take. Some of the clergy, because of their own ambivalence about the issue or because of their predilection to intellectualize every ethical decision, pushed for a year of discussion on the matter. Others of us maintained that the best education we could have was involvement (our time, energy, and money) with the problem. Our mentor was Bonhoeffer (not for his stand on abortion but his faith in action), who said, "We will not know what we will not do." This maxim was underscored by the immediacy of the subject with which we were dealing. The issue was not a "problem" but a *person,* a pregnant woman, growing more pregnant every day. If we clergy could afford the extravagance of discussion groups, workshops, and national conferences on abortion, she could not. Her choices were narrowed by her condition, and her condition would brook no prolonged theologizing about *her issue.* The decision was, therefore, to move ahead rapidly, keeping our "formal" education in this to a minimum and agreeing that our enlightenment on the subject would come from the day-to-day dealing with women who were presently suffering from an unjust law.

Although a few of us had been involved in referring women on an individual basis for abortion, we were for the most part almost totally ignorant about the subject. Shortly after Moody came to Judson Church in the fall of 1956, a former minister at Judson sent a woman from Florida to New York in search of an abortion. She was thirty-six years old, an active church woman, mother of three children, and presently separated from her husband. She felt that if the pregnancy were discovered, her marriage would be destroyed. Obviously there were no grounds for a "therapeutic abortion" in New York. Moody called up a layman in the church who had some experience with the problem; and like the blind leading the blind they struck out for New Jersey to run down the rumors of an "abortionist" who operated out of his house in West New York, New Jersey. They felt so ignorant and so frightened that when the nurse slammed the door in their faces because they did not have the code word, they were actually relieved. After following a half dozen false leads, a woman in the church found a group that operated out of a nice apartment house on the Upper West Side. After about three days the friend's pregnancy was terminated there for a low price of $600. It was a harrowing experience and was a portent of things to come over the next dozen years. Moody never forgot this first glimpse of that dark, ugly labyrinthian underground into which women were sent alone and afraid.

Self-education became our first order of business. In order to inform ourselves, we held several sessions with medical personnel, legal counsel, and psychiatrists.

Dr. Glenn Patterson, a member of Judson Church, had patients who had undergone illegal abortions, and he arranged for us to meet with several of those women to learn about their experiences and what help they felt would have been beneficial to them at that point in their lives.

That was the most important discussion we held since it provided insights into what needs women thought a clergy service should be prepared to meet. The women made it very clear that the last person in the world they would have gone to for help was the clergy because they believed, and they were probably right, that the role of the clergy in that situation would have been to talk them into having the baby. The second person that they would not talk to or turn to would have been their family doctor for much the same reasons; also, many felt the doctor would not keep their secret from other family members. We sensed that we were up against some long-standing historical biases which would make our job at best rather difficult. For our meeting with doctors we turned to those persons who had been publicly identified with the movement to reform abortion laws. Among those who participated was Dr. Robert Hall of Columbia Presbyterian Hospital, a longtime supporter of reform, who had written in the field and had certainly performed therapeutic abortions in his hospital. His counsel to the clergy as we gathered to talk about our resolve to establish a CCS (Clergy Consultation Service on Abortion) was very interesting in that it was far more cautionary than the action we had already decided to undertake. Dr. Hall felt we should do nothing "illegal" but instead should bring pressure to bear upon the hospitals to do so-called legal abortions. Since his hospital did a certain number of abortions, he felt that if all other hospitals did an equal number, this would gradually change the attitudes of other physicians. Dr. Hall recommended that we send pregnant women for hospital abortions in order to give hospital staffs an idea of the dimensions of the problem, even if not one woman was in fact aborted. The response of the clergy was that in addition to delaying a woman beyond the stage where it might be more dangerous to obtain even an illegal abortion, to "use" a woman in this fashion might do irreparable damage to her psyche. Thus we decided not to follow Dr. Hall's advice at all.

Another physician demonstrated the actual medical procedure, using a pelvic model and instruments. This man was not an Ob/Gyn but a pathologist who had a deep interest in the subject and was a longtime supporter of the right of a woman to have an abortion. The day the clergy went to "medical school" was a memorable one. The meeting was held at Judson Church, and the doctor brought all his instruments and the life-size model of the pelvic region including the cervix and the vagina. The nervous jokes and incredulous questions made it fairly obvious that we had majored in theology and not biology. One factor that kept the meeting from deteriorating into a stag party atmosphere was the presence of a woman Methodist minister from Staten Island, who had been associated with us from the beginning. The doctor then went step by step through the procedure which at that time was a D and C (dilation and curettage). In this procedure the cervix is dilated and the uterus is scraped with a curette so that the products of conception are removed from the woman's uterus. In describing the technique, he indicated when and what kind of pain would be felt by the woman. It was a "first" for all of us, and it proved in time to be one of the most valuable lessons we had. In the days of real ignorance about abortion when our images came from movies like *Alfie,* it was important for a counselor to describe to a woman what would happen to her in the procedure. It is a safe guess that the kind of preparation that doctor gave us for our counseling task surpassed anything the clergy had received in pastoral counseling courses.

Our legal advice came from the New York Civil Liberties Union. Aryeh Neier, who was then the Executive Director, and Ephraim London, a cooperating attorney and member of the Board of Directors of the N.Y.C.L.U., were the two people who counseled and advised us about what they believed would happen if we went ahead; they outlined the legal risk we would be taking if we pursued this course.

The N.Y.C.L.U. had already taken a strong stand on abortion and was 100 percent behind us. Ephraim London seemed to feel that if we clergy would function responsibly and somewhat conservatively in relation to the law, we might be able to accomplish our goals without being prosecuted. The cautionary notes laid down for us during those meetings were eventually built into the standard operating procedure of the CCS in the months to come. This standard operating procedure would become the clergy's working covenant and serve as a model for future Services in the rest of the country. What this meant was that we would only refer women to licensed gynecologists practicing outside the state of New York, where the law was prohibitory. The reason London gave for doing this was that should any prosecutions come about as a result of our referring women for abortions, having diverse jurisdictions involved would make it much more difficult to prosecute the clergy. It was at one and the same time both a way around the law and a precaution in the event we discovered we were, indeed, transgressing the law.

The legal advice which gave us the most assurance was Mr. London's recommendation that we never either assume or admit that we were breaking the law. At all times we were to behave as though we were acting within the laws of New York State and that as clergy we were bound to follow a higher moral law. Our standard public response, later, to all questions about the legality of our actions was that we were not in a position to determine the legality. The courts would have to make that determination.

Ephraim London's caution, which never included any "guarantee" that we would not be arrested, encouraged an openness about what we were planning to do. He firmly believed, and later events would bear him out, that everything we did needed to be done publicly. In other words, anything that gave the CCS the appearance of being clandestine would only serve to mitigate against what we hoped to accomplish. We took that advice to heart because it was not only good legal advice, but it was also good strategic advice.

At one memorable meeting we held with our lawyers, the clergy were laughing and joking about being arrested, nervous laughter though it was. As we talked about our feelings surrounding this unknown step on the road to civil disobedience, we agreed that if one of us got arrested, all the others would go along. Our solidarity stemmed from our conviction that to go ahead was in effect an act of conscience.

How our countenances fell when we expressed that solidarity to our lawyer and he replied that while it might be true that we would all like to "go" together, the district attorney would decide which *one* of us would be arrested. The rest of us might pray and be concerned about that individual, but there was no way we could force the authorities into a mass arrest.

At this point Moody agreed to become the spokesman for the CCS, to provide the direction and leadership necessary. This decision was based on the trust of the other clergy that when sudden decisions had to be made, that information would reach them quickly and they would follow whatever new instructions were issued. The group voluntarily placed considerable authority and confidence in the spokesman; they hoped that their faith in Moody, who would work closely with the legal and medical people, was not misplaced.

What emerged from that feeling of solidarity was an understanding of our mutual danger and the need to spell out very carefully a procedural covenant which would bind us together. The result was a standard operating procedure—verbal because we feared to put anything in writing—which included certain rules we would not, under any circumstances, violate. It was understood that each of us would counsel women in our own way; that is, the method we used would be the same method used in all of our pastoral counseling. However, the way in which a woman would be referred and to whom she would be referred would be agreed upon and cleared by the group. In this area there would be *no* room for individual preferences, nor was there room for individuality with respect to legal advice and protecting the privacy of the woman. On the whole we did not lay down very many rules for ourselves, but those we did make became part of our covenant and we could not easily break them without being expelled from the CCS.

We are sure that many thought our legal advisor was uptight and conservative. When we wanted to take a new chance or a more radical step, London's somber advice to us was, "Remember, you can't help those women who need assistance if you're in jail and the Service is closed down." He was right of course, and we heeded his advice for we believed that his priorities were correct; the challenging of the law was secondary to helping women get abortions.

At the end of our self-education project during which we met with a variety of people who contributed to our knowledge, we were faced with a very important decision, namely, what we would call ourselves. This led to a prolonged debate within the group. We did not disagree that we were taking on the role of consultants to women who were trying to make a decision over whether to carry an unplanned pregnancy to term. Thus we decided that the "Clergy Consultation Service" sounded like a good and appropriate name. What we could not decide on for a time was whether or not we should call ourselves a "Clergy Consultation Service *on Abortion*." It is important to remember that as late as 1967 "abortion" was a taboo word rarely used except in whispered conversations. Certainly people were aware that women had abortions, but still the word was not used in public debates or formal discussions. The question before us was whether or not to use the "unspoken word" in our name and thus run the risk of antagonizing some segments of the public by use of this emotionally loaded word or whether to settle for a euphemism like "problem pregnancy." The latter term would have softened the whole question about what we were doing as clergy and perhaps would have made it publicly more acceptable. Some of the clergy preferred "problem pregnancy" because it seemed less like flouting our intentions in the faces of our adversaries. Others of us preferred to use "abortion" because we hoped that by doing so we would be helping to "surface" the problem and open it up for public discussion; we even half-heartedly hoped using the word would help redeem both the word and the practice. The most persuasive argument and the one which ultimately convinced us that we should call ourselves the "Clergy Consultation Service on Abortion" (CCS) had to do with our reason for being and the people we wanted to serve. If we had not used "abortion" in our name, the women we wanted to reach might not have sought us out. A "Clergy Consultation Service on *Problem Pregnancies*" might have led women to think that we were available to help them bring their pregnancies to term and could have frightened off those desperate women we wanted to assist. "Abortion" clarified what we were about. The other side of that argument was that by using "abortion" we would create another misunderstanding, namely, that the only thing we were consulting about was abortion. In actual fact we had already decided that we were going to talk with women about all alternatives open to them: having and keeping the baby, giving it up for adoption, or having an abortion.

We did finally agree that we would rather be misunderstood by the public than avoided by women in trouble, and so the Clergy Consultation Service on Abortion was born. In later years Clergy Services in other states would choose to call themselves "Clergy Consultation Service on Problem Pregnancies," but by that time the public image of what we had done had been solidly established, and women everywhere in the United States turned to their local clergy service for help and reassurance.

Our next major hurdle was trying to discover the mechanics of organizing a public counseling service in an area where there were no precedents and no guidelines for us to follow. We were blazing new paths and of course made a few mistakes along the way.

In retrospect it seems clear that the strategy for the organization of the CCS was heavily influenced by and based upon the fear of being arrested and prosecuted for the act we were about to perform. It is an interesting fact that this caution on our part shaped the structure of the Clergy Service. For example, one of our decisions was to have no identifiable place of business. There would be no office, no address for the CCS. Instead it would be diffused and dispersed among all ministers and rabbis counseling women with problem pregnancies. In order to accomplish this we arranged for a telephone answering service, which later became an electronic answering service, that would refer callers to a minister or rabbi who was part of the CCS.

A decision had to be made as to where to locate physically the telephone answering service, which was the only tangible object of the CCS. It was nothing but a little gray box, a recording device that answered the phone automatically and gave the caller instructions. Robert Pierce, a member of Judson Church, who worked at the National Council of Churches, felt that we could place it in his office at 475 Riverside Drive. We all thought that would be a grand ecumenical gesture, good for the CCS, and a wonderful place to have it in the event anything were to happen. While we were in the process of having the phone installed, we received word from the legal counsel for the National Council of Churches that housing the phone would be too much of a risk for them to take. Afterwards we received a particularly sympathetic letter from a woman executive at the National Council expressing her deep regret that the council was unable to contribute to our effort in even this small way and offering her own support for the work we were about to do.

Of necessity we had the answering machine installed at Judson Church, which later turned out to be the ideal place for it since it was close to the spokesman and the staff who could change the taped message at a moment's notice if and when emergencies arose. The taped message gave the names and phone numbers of counselors available during a given week and women would then call for an appointment which would be kept at the church or synagogue with which the counselor was affiliated. This eliminated the need for a central office where women could be easily identified, detected, and possibly prosecuted, as even the clergy might have been if all counseling and referral had taken place in one location. By decentralizing the CCS, clergy were counseling in their own offices, and abortion counseling was just an additional pastoral responsibility, part of the natural order of their working lives.

Because of our caution we decided not to have any formal organization, no presidents or secretaries or officers of any kind. We also chose not to have any bank account in the name of the CCS. All of our funds were handled through Judson Church. We had been warned by our legal advisors that no money should ever pass between counselee and counselor. Historically women had been financially exploited due to the illicit nature of the practice, and any taint of profit to clergy would have been "anathema," reducing our credibility as honestly concerned citizens who had no personal stake in the abortion issue. Clearly we believed that not having a formal organization and not having a bank account protected us to some extent against legal prosecution.

The last act of our consciousness-raising program was to put down our statement of purpose that was the articulation and distillation of many lengthy discussions and numerous meetings. This document was the foundation from which we launched our service and on which we took our stand. That document must be read in order to understand our professional role in this social crisis and how we used that role in the service of this need.

CLERGY STATEMENT ON ABORTION LAW REFORM
AND
CONSULTATION SERVICE ON ABORTION

The present abortion laws require over a million women in the United States each year to seek illegal abortions which often cause severe mental anguish, physical suffering, and unnecessary death of women. These laws also compel the birth of unwanted, unloved, and often deformed children; yet a truly human society is one in which the birth of a child is an occasion for genuine celebration, not the imposition of a penalty or punishment upon the mother. These laws brand as criminals wives and mothers who are often driven as helpless victims to desperate acts. The largest percentage of abortion deaths are found among the 35-39-year-old married women who have five or six children. The present abortion law in New York is most oppressive of the poor and minority groups. A 1965 report shows that 94% of abortion deaths in New York City occurred among Negroes and Puerto Ricans.

We are deeply distressed that recent attempts to suggest even a conservative change in the New York State abortion law, affecting only extreme cases of rape, incest, and deformity of the child, have met with such immediate and hostile reaction in some quarters, including the charge that all abortion is "murder." We affirm that there is a period during gestation when, although there may be *embryo* life in the fetus, there is no living *child* upon whom the crime of murder can be committed.

Therefore we pledge ourselves as clergymen to a continuing effort to educate and inform the public to the end that a more liberal abortion law in this state and throughout the nation be enacted.

In the meantime women are being driven alone and afraid into the underworld of criminality or the dangerous practice of self-induced abortion. Confronted with a difficult decision and the means of implementing it, women today are forced by ignorance, misinformation, and desperation into courses of action that require humane concern on the part of religious leaders. Belief in the sanctity of human life certainly demands helpfulness and sympathy to women in trouble and concern for living children, many of whom today are deprived of their mothers, who die following self-induced abortions or those performed under sub-medical standards.

We are mindful that there are duly licensed and reputable physicians who in their wisdom perform therapeutic abortions which some may regard as illegal. When a doctor performs such an operation motivated by compassion and concern for the patient, and not simply for monetary gain, we do not regard him as a criminal, but as living by the highest standards of religion and of the Hippocratic oath.

Therefore believing as clergymen that there are higher laws and moral obligations transcending legal codes, we believe that it is our pastoral responsibility and religious duty to give aid and assistance to all women with problem pregnancies. To that end we are establishing a Clergymen's Consultation Service on Abortion which will include referral to the best available medical advice and aid to women in need.

Surfacing the Unspeakable

Unless one remembers the climate of opinion in those "dark days" of women's unliberation, one cannot easily understand the aura of silence and ignorance that hung over the subject of abortion. It is even more difficult to appreciate the lengthy discussion we had on how to announce what the clergy were about to do, publicly and officially.

We recognized that one of the risks connected with what we were about to do, given the uncertainty of its legality, was that the press in their need to get a story, and perhaps to put someone on the hot seat, could be in direct conflict with our own goals. Experience in other areas of social involvement had taught us that if all of us were allowed to speak on this delicate matter it was more likely that the CCS would be exposed in an unfavorable light. The media, even if sympathetic, could, by incorrectly stating our purpose or using the wrong language, state our case in an unhelpful way. Possibly we were overly sensitive about public relations, and perhaps this is why we were considered by others in the movement to be conservative. However, we believed that what we needed was the sympathy of the general public, who, even while feeling that abortion was wrong, were happy to see women, who were going that route anyway, receive assistance from a group of responsible people. We wanted to take with us in this venture as much public support as we could, even if it was only silent support. So the light in which this organization came to the attention of the public was, we believed, tremendously important for its future.

The clergy spent long sessions discussing just how we would publicly surface the CCS. One of the traditional ways this is done is by holding a press conference. After examining this alternative, we decided against it because to hold a press conference on an issue as delicate as abortion was at that time could have been devastating. One determined, antagonistic reporter can make any group look very bad if he wants to. Since we could not possibly know in advance which reporter would be sent by which newspaper or television station, we were unwilling to risk being questioned by one who was anti-abortion.

Another way to "go public" is to gradually leak the news in a variety of places—a radio show here, a television show there, an item in a newspaper story. After consideration we rejected that alternative because it was what our legal advisors had cautioned us against, namely, the appearance of being an underground, somewhat secret organization. To have leaked our existence bit by bit would have created the impression that we had something to hide. So it was decided that we would announce our existence by way of an exclusive story given to Edward B. Fiske, religion editor of the *New York Times*. On May 22, 1967, a front-page story headlined "Clergymen Offer Abortion Advice: 21 Ministers and Rabbis Form New Group—Will Propose Alternatives" appeared.

Though Fiske was never present at any of our discussions of what we wanted to accomplish in the first public announcement of the CCS, his article was a superb media interpretation of our aims and goals. Long after, we credited that opening announcement as responsible for setting the tone for the CCS. It made our actions acceptable to many people who otherwise might have thought this to be the work of wild-eyed radicals breaking the law.

At the present time it does not seem very radical that twenty-one ministers and rabbis were going to establish a counseling service for the sole purpose of advising women with problem pregnancies, but in the late sixties such an activity was quite a departure from the traditional roles clergy were usually seen as playing. We were very apprehensive about the reaction this announcement might bring from both the public at large and the law enforcement agencies. We had considered raising the question of our "legality" with the local district attorney's office, prior to opening, but our legal counsel advised us against doing anything of the sort. Ephraim London felt that any premature contact with law enforcement would ultimately be to our disadvantage, and so no contact was made.

Instead we decided to be absolutely open about our aims, intentions, and goals, stating those as explicitly as we could in order to mitigate against any appearance of an underground or illicit activity. We also interpreted our actions so that they would be seen as an extension of our pastoral responsibility toward this need of women, which was more prevalent than any of us had imagined.

Our apprehension concerning the police was confirmed a few days after the CCS opened when we found that our phones at the church were being tapped. It was not the electronic answering service that was being tapped but the regular telephones of Judson Memorial Church. We tended to take this report very seriously because the tip came from the police department itself. As a direct result of this report we never discussed any CCS business of consequence on the church lines; instead we made all important calls from a pay phone some blocks away from the church. In order to deal with incoming calls from the clergy (in the beginning we ran to the public phone and called the clergy counselor back), we developed a cryptic language based on abbreviations and associations which most lay people, and we hoped the wiretappers, would not understand. Of course, as time passed, our paranoia decreased, and we became emboldened to the point where on occasion we would actually mention one of our "abortionists" by name on the church phones.

Another concern we faced in the beginning was just what the response of women would be. This concern was quickly dissipated as the phones rang incessantly that first week, and we began to see the outline of the dimensions of the issue that was there in our society. Far more women responded to our offer of advice and counsel than we ever dreamed were out there in our city. Calls were coming from every state in the Union, and women were willing to travel great distances just for a counseling session and information.

Before opening the Service we had reached a decision regarding our own anticipated paranoia concerning the women who would come to us for counseling. We agreed that we would have to strike a balance between occasional suspicion and irresponsible laxity. Feeling fairly sure that it would be hard to detect a "ringer" or police plant who came to see us, it would have been a real disservice to expose *all* counselees to *our* fear at a time when they were having to cope with their own anxiety about going through a criminalizing process. Our problems would have become part of their burden. So we decided not to insist that women tell us their true names; even when we had our doubts, we would not ask to see any identification. Obviously this practice meant that a police-woman seeking evidence for the authorities to prosecute the CCS could go through the Service and be referred like anyone else. As far as we know, since we never had any legal trouble, this never happened.

But we did have close and unsettling calls from time to time. Lyle Guttu, one of our clergy, told us of a couple he had counseled who had returned to thank him after the wife's abortion was finished. The man was so grateful that he wanted Pastor Guttu to feel free to call him if he could ever be of help in his line of work. Asked what his line of work was, he replied that he was a captain in the New York City Police Department. So we did have our dealings with the police, but usually it was in the context of helping them. As part of the general population, their wives, daughters, and friends would from time to time need help like anyone else.

Seeing the evidence of this overwhelming problem, in the second week of our existence we put out a call to the allied professions, particularly doctors and psychiatrists, to come forward and help us in this work that we were doing. In our statement we said, "This one long parade of mental anguish and physical suffering is but symbolic of the immeasurable number of human beings that are in dire need of even the kind of limited help which this service can give. This social problem is like an iceberg. Great chunks of human pain and desperation are all beneath the surface. It can only be met by doctors and psychiatrists who courageously step forward to help reinterpret the law so as to bring light and hope to the thousands of people who suffer—usually in quiet, and sometimes in death—the miseries and heartbreak of backstreet abortions."

We very quickly learned that the medical profession was not really concerned about helping with this problem. We had had intimations of this in our first week of counseling. Woman after woman told us that when she thought she might be pregnant she went immediately to her gynecologist for help only to receive a most callous and almost indifferent response. Some of these women had been under the care of the same gynecologist for five, ten, or fifteen years, and they were rightfully shocked when their own physicians abruptly ended the discussion with the statement that they could not help in any way.

Despite the negative reports which we received from some of the women we had counseled that first week of our existence, we issued our call to the medical profession on the assumption that like any profession or group, there would be some who would respond to a call for help. But there were none. Not only were physicians unwilling to assist the clergy who were, after all, dealing with what was clearly a medical problem, but many in the medical profession also put obstacles in our way as we attempted to do a responsible job. One of the few demands we made on the women seeking our assistance was that they bring to their consultation with the clergy a dated note from their doctor indicating that they had received both a pelvic examination and pregnancy test and were so many weeks of gestation. In order to make a responsible referral, it was essential that the rabbi or minister have this crucial information. If the doctors would provide us with this information, we felt we would be on some sort of firm ground in fulfilling our professional counseling task. It seemed a small enough request to make of the medical profession, especially since it was their patients we were going to help. However, most doctors refused even this minimal assistance to their patients, fearing perhaps that to do so would somehow incriminate them or give them reputations as doctors who would refer women for "illegal" abortions. This refusal to give a note did not come from every doctor, but from a clear majority. In time, we developed a form letter which we sent to physicians who had refused to provide a patient with the necessary note. Incredible as it may seem, our letter began with an explanation of why the clergy required the pregnancy note in the first place. Here is an excerpt from that letter:

First, it was found that women's memories were often unreliable, and the length of pregnancy, as I'm sure you understand, determines what options are available to her. The second reason we require the internal examination and note is that we assume doctors will make their patients aware of any unusual medical problems that may exist which would make termination difficult or unsafe.

What we have discovered, to our shock and regret, is that physicians who are very willing to refer their patients to us as well as see them post-operatively refuse for reasons we fail to understand to provide them with a note that they would willingly write for an employer or a school. We are quite willing to continue handling problem pregnancies until doctors themselves are ready to deal effectively with what is, after all, a medical problem. However, we are upset when physicians refuse to cooperate in such a small way and we fail to see any possible harm that could come to a doctor. As a consequence, the woman is forced to undergo a second examination by a cooperative physician, thereby incurring additional expenses at a time when she can least afford it.

We do hope that you will reconsider and help your patients at least to the extent of providing them with the necessary verification.

Continuous refusal of a majority of doctors to help women who had been their patients for years convinced us that many of them had their own problems regarding a woman's right to control her own destiny. Perhaps we are mistaken, but it is our impression that this judgment by the medical profession was eroded as increasing numbers of women sought assistance from the CCS and the Service itself received wider publicity. By the time we disbanded the New York CCS in 1970, more than 50 percent of all women we saw were referred to us by their personal physician.

Another concern we had as we opened the CCS was that the Catholic Church and a certain portion of the public would be upset and consequently respond negatively to our organization. So we were all pleasantly surprised by the largely positive response and the relatively minor negative comment on the service we were offering.

If the Roman Catholic Church was deeply disturbed by our counseling program, it did not make this known openly. We tried to be respectful of opposing points of view. In the first year of the Service, we appeared on numerous occasions in debates with clergy of the Roman Catholic Church. A favorite opponent in those early days of the CCS was a professor from Boston University Law School, Father Robert Drinan, later to become a congressman from his district in Massachusetts. He never knew the influential role he played in developing the theological and legal position CCS finally took on the abortion issue.

At the International Conference on Abortion in Washington, D.C., September 6-8, 1967, which was sponsored by the Kennedy Foundation in cooperation with Harvard University, a number of moral theologians and medical leaders met to present papers. It was a very conservative group of persons that came out against the liberalization of the law. Among them was Rev. Robert F. Drinan, S.J. His paper was called "The Right of the Fetus to Be Born," and for the most part it was a thoroughly orthodox presentation of the Roman Catholic Church's position. But being a philosopher of jurisprudence and a professor of law, he was also interested in the laws regarding abortion; so, within the body of this very conservative paper, there was an incredible defense of the case for *repeal* of the abortion law as opposed to the popular *compromise* of a reform law supported by the American Law Institute. To have a Roman Catholic theologian of Drinan's stature writing an incredibly convincing argument for *repeal* as over against *reform* was a real boost in the battle ahead. In that paper Drinan said, among other arguments:

> Abortion on request—or an absence of law with respect to abortion—has at least the merit of not involving the law and society in the business of selecting those persons whose lives may be legally terminated. A system of permitting abortion on request has the undeniable virtue of neutralizing the law so that while the law does not forbid abortion, it does not on the other hand sanction it—even on presumably restructured basis. [The law] neither concedes nor denies the individuals the right to abort their unborn children. It leaves the area unregulated in the same way that the law abstains from regulating many areas of conduct where moral issues are involved.

It was surely the influence of men like Father Drinan, John Courtney Murray, and Cardinal Cushing that softened the Catholic reaction to the opening of the CCS. Progress was real because less than twenty years prior to that time Margaret Sanger had been barred from speaking in the First Congregational Church in Holyoke, Massachusetts, on the threat of economic reprisal by the Roman Catholic Church to lay members of that Protestant church.

This was the first indication we had of the unspoken acceptance of abortion itself and the widespread tolerance for women seeking to undergo the procedure. While abortion, at that time, was not ordinarily a topic of conversation, we sensed a very broad concern for the welfare of women. Since it was understood that women were going to get abortions, the only valid question became where and under what conditions. If someone, in this case the clergy, was trying to be responsible in relationship to this problem by helping women find at least a modicum of dignity and decent medical care, that person was to be applauded and not denigrated.

The fact that the counselors were clergy was not an unimportant aspect of public acceptance. One of the many letters we received that first week stated simply, "I don't believe in God, but each time I read about courageous efforts by men of the cloth to put human values above dogma or antiquated laws, I realize that there is an essential unity among men on earth." It is difficult now to believe that someone would refer to the clergy efforts as "courageous" for simply counseling a woman in need. However, to realize certain risks were involved, one needs to recall that the New York law in 1967 read that one could receive a one-thousand-dollar fine and up to one year in prison for aiding and abetting a woman in attaining an abortion. The clergy felt that they were doing what was required of them. However, some of our counselors joined without the consent of their congregations and were later reprimanded for their involvement.

Most letters, however, were much like the one from a public health nurse who considered the CCS, ". . . an ingenious idea. You are offering a much needed humanitarian service." Her letter was to prove prophetic, for it concluded by suggesting, "Perhaps your action will serve as a demonstration for the rest of the country." One of the very few critical letters expressed the view: "The most horrendous thing about abortion is that the life being destroyed has no right to defend itself. . . . Perhaps you would have us throw out the Ten Commandments simply because they are difficult for some people to obey." This was a forerunner of the argument later refined by the Catholic Church which claimed in no uncertain terms that abortion is murder.

One of the earliest practical problems with which we needed to cope was how to find those doctors who were willing to perform "illegal" abortions. Without those resources we were of no value to women. When the CCS opened, we were able to refer to one or two to whom several of us had individually sent patients over the years. However, we did obtain from the women who sought us out leads about other abortionists whose names were unfamiliar to us. Often a woman came merely to find out what we knew about a doctor whose name had been passed along to her, whether the doctor was qualified and still in practice. If we had no information in our files on a particular "physician," we would actively check him out, developing as time passed an almost routine procedure.

The first fact we needed to determine was whether or not the name we had was that of a real person or whether it was an assumed name. We never pursued any abortionist operating under an assumed name since there was no foolproof way to check on the medical license of a "physician" operating under a pseudonym. One of the strictures laid down by our attorneys at the outset was that patients be referred by the CCS only to licensed physicians, preferably gynecologists, and so the checking of credentials was absolutely necessary.

While we would have preferred qualified gynecologists, our norm in those days was a licensed physician with experience. Given a choice between a gynecologist who had never performed an abortion and an ordinary physician who had, we usually preferred the physician with demonstrated skill. Long before there was talk of paraprofessionals performing abortions, we realized that a physician who over the years had performed hundreds of D & C's was often better qualified than a gynecologist who performed perhaps one therapeutic D & C a year in his hospital.

On one occasion that we know of we were duped into believing someone was a licensed physician, having been assured of this fact by his famous colleague. Since the women we referred to these doctors had no postoperative complications, we had no reason to doubt his credentials. Not until the police arrested both of them in Washington, D.C., did we learn that he was a totally untrained Mexican national, with a lot of talent!

Once we established that a reputed abortionist was in fact a physician living and practicing openly in a community, we would make contact.

Posing as a pregnant woman, one of our staff would make a phone call to the physician and set up an appointment, using prearranged code words if necessary. The staff member would keep the appointment, maintaining the illusion of a woman with an unwanted pregnancy. However, often times we did not get beyond the front door because the doctor's office was either located in a badly rundown area or because the entryway was obviously filthy. Our visual impression was often decisive, believing as we did that a woman should not have to put up with unsanitary or unsafe conditions. One memorable visit made to a well-known New Jersey abortionist (fee: $600) was a dead end because his abortion office was situated in a house in the heart of a slum area. In his filthy waiting room, packed with about thirty prospective patients, chipped paint was falling from the ceiling onto a floor which appeared not to have been washed in weeks. Upon leaving, one could not help but notice the black Cadillac with MD license plates parked in front of the house. Later we learned and verified that he had an elegant office for his regular patients in another community. Many of the abortionists we knew of did not seem to plow back any of their profits into their illicit practices. If the neighborhood and waiting room were acceptable, the staff member would, still posing as a pregnant patient, actually see the doctor and explain the fabricated situation. She maintained the deception with the doctor long enough to get an impression of his manner with patients first (was he warm and friendly, or cool, gruff, and condescending?) and then to elicit from him a description of the medical procedure he used in performing abortions as well as the fee being charged. If his personality was pleasing and the technique was one which our medical advisors considered acceptable (they were adamantly against "packing" as well as the use of general anesthesia in an office setting), the staff member would reveal the "patient's" true identity and produce a note from the CCS authorizing her to speak on the organization's behalf.

Our opposition to the "packing" procedure was inflexible. This technique requires the insertion of some materials into the uterus, and theoretically, at least, within twenty-four hours the patient should have a spontaneous abortion. Aside from the fact that it was undependable (i.e., did not always work), the danger of infection was too great for us to recommend names of practitioners of that technique. The fear of general anesthesia came from our medical advisors' belief that it should always be administered under hospital conditions. One of our advisors often said that if a member of his own family were scheduled for surgery, the credentials he would check most carefully would be those of the anesthesiologist. On that basis we used only doctors who gave local anesthetics and we chose physicians who used no anesthesia over ones who used general anesthesia in an office setting.

Only once did we meet an abortionist who had heard of the Clergy Service and was not anxious to receive our referrals. A well-known Philadelphia abortionist literally threw us out of his office after being told of our CCS connection and shouted as he slammed the door in our face, "The clergy are big trouble!"

All other abortionists were perfectly willing to work out a relationship with the CCS that protected both themselves and the patients and for which a fair fee was established. A fair fee in 1967 was $600; in 1970 when we disbanded, it was $300; in 1972 under a liberal abortion law in New York it was $125. Information about this new contact was then reported back to the clergy, who in consultation with our medical advisors, would decide whether or not to monitor the physician.

Our monitoring technique was simple and dependable since the patients themselves did it for us. When a new doctor was tentatively "approved," only one member of the CCS was authorized to make referrals to him. That minister or rabbi would urge every woman who saw the doctor to report back, either in person or by mail, any discrepancies between what she had been told to expect and what actually occurred. Was the medical and psychological treatment satisfactory? Was she charged the price told her by the clergy? Monitoring on a limited basis meant that the doctor could not tell us one thing and do something entirely different to the patient without running the risk of losing our goodwill. After three or four weeks, if we received consistently satisfactory reports from the women, information about this new "resource" would be shared with all of the other members of the CCS.

From that point on the monitoring would be done by all the clergy, who during all the "illegal" years requested every woman to let us know when she returned how things had gone and that she was OK. A surprisingly high percentage (40 percent) of all counselees did recontact their counselor after the abortion, providing us with a steady stream of information about the doctors we were using. As soon as we discovered a serious complication, repeated reports of mistreatment or overcharges, we would drop the doctor without giving him any advance warning.

Lest anyone assume that this was harsh treatment of a humanitarian operating outside the law and risking incarceration in order to help desperate women, consider the advantage to the doctors of working with the Clergy Service. The clergy were able to do for them something which had not been done before, namely, refer to them a steady volume of patients who had been examined, screened, and counseled in advance. This meant that only patients without medical contraindications were referred; also these patients arrived with a certain sophistication about and understanding of what was in store for them, having had their fears allayed and a detailed explanation of the medical procedure provided by their clergy-counselor. Contrast this clientele with that ordinarily seen by most "illegal" abortionists—women who knew nothing about what they were about to go through, women whose fear and anxiety often made it impossible to perform the abortion—and the benefits of working with us become clear.

One of the greatest advantages to the abortionists was a reduction in their own fear of being exposed or turned in by a patient. Having gone through the CCS meant there was less risk that the woman was a police operative and this factor made the doctors feel more secure.

Under these circumstances we had no hesitation about dropping a doctor who blatantly violated our understanding. Usually within several days the doctor would be on the phone wondering why we had stopped sending patients. If our only complaints had to do with overcharging, we would usually give him another chance if he promised to stand by the agreed-upon fee.

The doctor with whom we had the longest relationship (two years) was also the source of much grief. Working with him in his Puerto Rican office was a lab technician who ran tests on patients prior to the abortion. For this service there was a separate charge of $10. The doctor's fee was at first $500 and then at our request dropped to $400 and finally $350. While we never had complaints about the doctor overcharging our women, we would periodically receive reports that the technician was charging patients anywhere up to $30. At the start of our relationship we would cut the doctor off from referrals; he would call, and we would explain the problem; the technician's fee would drop back to $10. Later on we would just call the doctor and ask him to deal with the technician.

In speculating about why we were more tolerant of the weaknesses in this situation, the only explanation we could give was that he was one of the few abortionists who dealt with us in a purely professional manner. He never attempted to ingratiate himself with us nor did he ever hint that he would "like to make a contribution to the church," which so many of the others had offered to do, an offer we always refused. On our last visit to San Juan, we accidentally learned that our favorite doctor was the proud owner of a string of race horses worth almost a million dollars. Think of the churches we might have built!

After the first weeks, media curiosity about the CCS mushroomed. While we were always open about counseling and referring, we refused to provide the media with the more intimate details of our organization. It was our belief that we had an obligation to protect the anonymity of two sources: the women who were going through abortions and the doctors who were performing them illegally. Both the women and the doctors would have been placed in jeopardy if we had enabled the press to give them any publicity at all. This created from the earliest days a clear conflict between the aggressive reporter who wanted to get a story and the clergy who in order to serve women responsibly needed to protect both doctors and counselees.

Probably because we were uncooperative, a reporter from the *New York Post* posed as a pregnant woman and came to us for counseling. She intended to do an exposé of the CCS, not with any intention of hurting us but rather in order to give us wider exposure. This occurred during the first few weeks of our existence, long before we believed the CCS well enough established to withstand the pressures that might be brought by our opponents who could use her article as evidence of our "illegal" activity. After learning of the story from a friend, we decided to do all we could to have it suppressed. With that goal in mind we asked a friend to intercede with the publisher of the *Post*. The inner counsels of that newspaper finally decided that the story would be detrimental to what the clergy were trying to do and so it was killed. We were very grateful to the *New York Post* and hoped that it viewed the situation as the workings of a responsible newspaper rather than the suppression of freedom of the press.

Although we felt that story would have harmed us, it is an illustration of the way in which people wanted to help. There were always persons who advised us to get lots of publicity, but we usually shunned this advice. We had decided very early in the game that our primary function was the counseling of women and remembered our lawyer's warning: "You won't be able to help women if you're in jail."

Our unwillingness to risk overexposure by giving stories to the press, appearing on radio and television, accompanying women going for abortions, etc., eventually caused us to be labeled "conservatives" by allies in the struggle. Nevertheless, it was our conviction that if we could weather the early storms and problems we might encounter as we entered this uncharted area without tarnishing the image of the clergy as professional counselors, our success would be in the best interest of women seeking help.

The Making of a Model: A New Kind of Counseling Service

It is important to understand that back in the spring of 1967, we did not establish the New York Clergy Consultation Service with any plans, hopes, or designs (conscious or unconscious) for expanding into what it ultimately and accidentally became—a nationwide effort involving thousands of ministers and rabbis, which today includes growing numbers of lay counselors as well as priests and at least one nun. Ignorant of the national dimensions of the problem of unwanted pregnancies, we intended to tackle the problems of an unjust law in New York State and never thought as we began that the New York CCS would be duplicated elsewhere in the country.

So it was purely accidental that the model for a counseling service situated in New York could be easily copied. The makeup of the first CCS was influenced by our lawyers and our own strategic sense of what was both possible and practical. In retrospect it is easy to recognize that simplicity was the decisive factor in the duplication that followed. An observer looking at the CCS saw no office, no staff, no board of directors, no bank account, no trustees, just a paper organization with a telephone number and an electronic telephone answering machine serving thousands of women a year. Out of our own local needs we had established a helping agency which cost practically nothing to run. Our average expenses annually for the New York CCS were around $1,800, usually offset by contributions given by Judson Church or by grateful women after their abortion. All our procedures were designed to meet our own special needs, and to our surprise these procedures became the primary basis for the spread of Clergy Consultation Services to other areas of the country.

Late in 1967 the California Committee on Therapeutic Abortion asked Hugh Anwyl, who was then pastor of the Mt. Hollywood Congregational Church, to establish a Clergy Service in Los Angeles. Mr. Anwyl came to New York, and we shared with him our knowledge and what little experience we had already accumulated. He returned to Los Angeles where in May of 1968 the Clergy Counseling Service for Problem Pregnancies was established. With minor modifications, it was a facsimile of the New York CCS. By November, 1968, there was a CCS in New Jersey, and shortly thereafter one opened in Philadelphia.

Though we were not quite *deluged* by requests for information from clergy, we did receive queries from a substantial number, some of whom ultimately went on to develop Clergy Services in their own areas. If we were to single out the major force which led to the mushrooming of CCS groups around the country, we would have to attribute it to a growing awareness of the number of women who needed help.

As was mentioned earlier, we had no way of anticipating or calculating in advance how many women would seek us out. Because abortion was "illegal," there were no reliable statistics available on the number of procedures performed. The figure most frequently quoted by abortion reformers was one million annually, but no one knew for sure. Due to our helpless ignorance, we were not prepared for the deluge. Our files bulged with letters from desperate women across this country who were perfectly willing to come to New York merely to consult with one of our clergy, knowing full well that their abortion would be performed in some other state or country. Other women called from all over the United States to make appointments for a consultation. During our first year of existence, we agreed to see any woman who could get to New York City.

However, as time passed, it became clear that the burden of the entire country was too great for the New York CCS to carry by itself, and a way to serve those non-New York women closer to their homes needed to be found. We briefly considered telephone referral for all nonresidents but discarded that idea quickly since it would have violated our belief in the desirability and necessity for face-to-face counseling. With the passage of time and with firsthand experience we had become wedded to this principle. There was no satisfactory substitute for *seeing* the women. One simply could not gather the same information during a phone conversation, and what we saw often affected our counseling. Fear cannot always be detected over the phone, but it is hard to miss in the eyes of a frightened young woman. Long-distance phone calls might mitigate against an extended conversation about the guilt associated with seeking an abortion, but conversation in the relaxed atmosphere of a counselor's office provided the woman with an opportunity to articulate her feelings. Most of the physical or even emotional problems that could be spotted in a moment if the woman is sitting across from you are impossible to detect over the phone. If the counselor made a referral by phone, he could not be certain of the length of a woman's pregnancy, a crucial factor in making a responsible referral; but when she came to see the counselor, she was required to bring a physician's note stating the length of her pregnancy in weeks.

This mandatory pre-counseling examination was initiated in reaction to a near tragedy some six months after we opened the New York CCS. Previously we had required only positive proof of pregnancy, and on that basis one of the young women we counseled was referred to a doctor in Puerto Rico. As a result of a variety of circumstances, including the fact that Donna was a minor whose parents could not afford the air fare to accompany her, she was taken to the doctor's office by one of our people who was visiting San Juan and checking out abortionists. Our person remained in the waiting room during the procedure. After an hour, she heard scurrying footsteps and anxious voices behind the door leading to the operating room. Also the waiting room was locked so no one could leave. Finally the doctor appeared, looking drawn, took our person aside, and said, "Well, she died." After what seemed like hours but must have only been moments, he continued, "But we saved her." Contrary to the information Donna had given us, her pregnancy was well into the fifteenth week, and she had experienced a fetal reaction to the anesthetic, so violent that her vital signs had momentarily stopped. She had been revived, but nevertheless a call was immediately placed to one of our medical advisors in New York, to whom the doctor explained what had happened and the course of treatment Donna was receiving. Our New York doctor approved, not learning until later that immediately afterwards the doctor in Puerto Rico asked whether he should try again to do the abortion since Donna was still pregnant.

Within hours of that incident, the New York CCS's tape-recorded message was modified to include the following:

> There is no charge for the consultation, but it will be necessary for women to bring along to the counselor a dated note from either an obstetrician or a gynecologist stating that you have had a pelvic examination and indicating in weeks the length of your pregnancy. No consultation will be possible without this prior examination, and the results of urine tests alone will not be acceptable.

By the following day all members of the New York CCS had been notified that no further referrals were to be made to that particular doctor in Puerto Rico. What we neither needed nor wanted was an abortionist who gambled with women's lives and would have permitted a lay person to determine whether an incomplete abortion should be repeated. It was a painfully hard way to learn.

Our final reason for rejecting telephone counseling had to do with our desire to lend the respectability of the church to the woman's decision, making personal contact with a supportive clergy counselor important. Telephone counseling clearly worked against our goals of making responsible referrals, alleviating fear and guilt, and being emotionally supportive to women.

The only other avenue that lay open to us to help women in distant places was to encourage and assist those clergy who had expressed interest in setting up a counseling service in their own states. At the same time we could actively enlist clergy in other states.

Our goal was to enable any woman to see a counselor within a reasonable distance from her home. By and large we called on friends who, like members of the New York CCS, were involved in social issues. We were lucky to have Spencer Parsons in Illinois, Harry Smith in North Carolina, and George Telford in Florida, among those who answered our call for help. Although we encouraged them to develop local Clergy Services, we never consciously put undue pressure on them. We didn't need to. That Clergy Services emerged under the leadership of these people was more a result of the pressure they began to feel as we referred local women to them for counseling. They soon discovered that they could not handle the load alone and began to enlist their colleagues' assistance.

During the summer of 1968 we were faced with a major

decision, namely, whether to establish an umbrella group to be called the "National Clergy Consultation Service on Abortion," which would then seek foundation support, or to continue along in our somewhat disorganized manner. The primary reason for establishing the National CCS was that it would provide travel funds for meetings with clergy around the country who were organizing Services and wanted detailed information about our experiences in New York. Indulging paranoia in our infancy, we never put anything on paper which could incriminate us, and consequently travel was an expensive necessity for which funds needed to be raised. Furthermore the growth of Clergy Consultation Services, especially at our urging, required that we provide them, in the beginning at least, with safe and secure medical resources which had been checked out. We hoped that as time passed and new groups were well established, they would be able to develop their own medical resources. When that happened, it would become National's function to keep an up-to-date negative list of practicing abortionists as well as a list of the doctors individual CCS's were referring to. Thus, for example, the Michigan CCS could call requesting information on a particular abortionist, and we could tell them whether he was on our negative list or whether another CCS was referring to him. If we had no information, they would then proceed to check him out. If the report came up negative, they would forget him; he would be added to our list of inferior abortionists. If another CCS was referring patients to him, it was generally understood that no referrals would be made without consulting with the CCS that had "discovered" him. This was important because often the doctor was handling as many patients as safety allowed. Another CCS referring women to him could mean that women would experience delays in getting appointments or the doctor would overburden himself, possibly providing poorer service. Having learned through trial and error that abortionists would often negotiate different arrangements with different Clergy Consultation Services so that a woman referred by the Massachusetts CCS might pay, to the same doctor, $50 or $100 more than a woman referred by the Connecticut CCS, we encouraged communication between Services hoping to avoid such situations.

Aware that bringing new Services into being would result in a brief period of dependency on the resources and experience of the New York CCS, we decided the needs could best be met by establishing yet another paper organization, the National CCS on Abortion. With a five-thousand-dollar grant from a philanthropist, the National Service was created in November, 1968. Like its local affiliates, it had no paid staff, no officers, no bank account. The continued concern of Judson Church meant that staff was allowed to give time to this new project, and office space at the church was made available. The donor later said that he never got such a good return on so small an investment.

The following spring the first annual meeting of all Clergy Consultation Service coordinators was held at Judson. There were perhaps a dozen people present, representing Services already public and those in formation. (By 1972 we had grown so large that three regional meetings were held in place of one national get-together.) We came together that first time to hammer out a policy concerning the relationship between National CCS and local groups and the relationship of local groups to one another. At that meeting decisions and directions were determined that have not substantially changed in the intervening years. National CCS would be a loose federation of Clergy Services, each with local autonomy. While National might on occasion make recommendations, all final policy decisions would be made locally. National would be a provider and enabler, and at times a persuader, but never a dictator of policies.

One of the serious temptations that we managed to resist was to create a large institution out of the National CCS which would have a national office, full-time staff, and large budget. We received a great deal of pressure to build this kind of structure, which we perceived would become a self-perpetuating bureaucracy that would eventually have to develop rationale and increased finances for its continued existence. Since we conceived of all clergy counseling as an interim task, we were fearful of what might become an empire-building, self-serving organization whose preservation would take priority even when its existence was no longer required. The price we had to pay in order to resist that institutional seduction was for Judson Church and the New York CCS to take more of the burden. The interim lasted longer than we had foreseen, but the principle of an ad hoc, low cost, voluntary national organization paid off. Power plays, "Parkinson's law," and political fighting over control of an "empire" were avoided. No one wanted to take over a thankless, voluntary task with heavy responsibility and few rewards.

Affiliation of local Clergy Consultation Services with National CCS was completely voluntary. All Services agreed on three requirements for affiliation, and they were essentially the same as the ground rules established by local Services. First, no Clergy Service affiliated with National would ever charge a fee for counseling and referral. In subsequent years, we discovered a handful of counselors around the country who violated this rule, and they were immediately dropped by the CCS they were working with. Several of the Clergy Services, when hard pressed financially, entertained the idea of charging a nominal fee, but none ever went beyond the point of encouraging contributions.

Second, all Clergy Services affiliated with National would provide person-to-person counseling. From time to time we would receive reports of telephone or group counseling, but as a national group we discouraged it. However, as years passed and lay counselors became a more visible part of the Clergy Services, some walk-in centers with group counseling were developed (usually in urban areas), but the vast majority of women are still seen individually.

Finally, no Clergy Service affiliated with National would have among its members any counselors who referred to non-approved resources. This rule has always been at the same time the hardest to enforce and the most important to follow. Probably every Clergy Service has had at least one member who for the best of reasons (closer, less expensive) has referred a woman to an abortionist who had not been checked out and approved. Each CCS developed its own style of dealing with wayward counselors. Allen Hinand handled one such case in Pennsylvania by calling the minister who had made an unapproved referral and asking him whether he was aware of having sent the woman to a gas station attendant who had never been anywhere near a medical school. Other Clergy Services were less inclined to direct confrontation and would simply "forget" to list the counselor's name on the tape recording which directed women to a minister or rabbi for assistance. When a member of the New York CCS violated our understanding, he was voted out of the Service by the membership.

Careful control over where women were sent was not a whimsical part of the covenant of each Clergy Service. Knowing the credentials and skills of an abortionist before referring patients was a prerequisite; in the absence of an ongoing relationship Clergy Services had no power to deal with an incompetent physician. Both problems are best illustrated by a situation which developed in the summer of 1968. We were contacted by three young women, all of whom had gone through the New York CCS, been counseled by the same rabbi, been referred to the same unapproved resource in New Jersey, gone for their abortions, paid their $450, and were all still pregnant. Each was beyond the stage where an office abortion could safely be performed and had no further financial resources to draw upon. The counselor who had made the referrals had left New York several weeks earlier for a position in the Midwest. We immediately contacted him requesting an explanation; at the same time we investigated the doctor, to whom the women had been referred. The "doctor" turned out not to be a physician, but was instead a guy who had made a deal with an actual doctor in New Jersey to "use" his office several days a week. The counselor who had made the referral knew that the doctor was licensed but never pursued the credentials of the man who was actually doing the abortions. Evidently the women who came to us reporting incomplete abortions had been the only ones referred to this resource by our counselor.

In the absence of a relationship with the bogus physician, we had no leverage and could not, officially at least, demand that he return the money to each of these women. Occasionally a woman we had referred to an "approved" resource would have an incomplete abortion. In those instances we would simply contact the physician in question, and all monies would be refunded to the patient. Before the establishment of CCS, such refunds were unheard of, but our relationship enabled us to successfully act as advocates for women since the doctors were anxious to stay in our good graces.

This nightmarish situation was resolved in a somewhat unorthodox way after the man posing as a physician had flatly refused to return the money to these women. We chose several of the strongest looking men at Judson Church and asked them to accompany one woman to his New Jersey office where, without making any direct threats, they let him know that they were not satisfied with his refusal. During their visit the man "changed his mind" and refunded the $450. The success of this mission was communicated to the other women who then followed the same course of nonviolent confrontation with the imposter and were similarly rewarded.

On the surface this incident may appear to have had a happy ending, but it didn't. Three women were still pregnant against their will, and as far as we know each carried her unwanted pregnancy to term. The outcome would have been different had they been referred to an approved resource.

At that first National CCS meeting, the relationship between local Clergy Services was never clearly articulated. Though it was understood that we were "all in this together" and that what threatened one Service threatened us all, a formal policy was never hammered out. Over the years there were points of conflict and disagreement between local Services as well as between local and the National Service. Yet at crucial moments, particularly when there were conflicts with the authorities, we all stuck together.

Bearing in mind that Clergy Services everywhere operated in a gray area of dubious legality, it is remarkable how few confrontations with the authorities there were. The first occurred in the spring of 1969 when the Reverend Robert W. Hare, pastor of the Congregation of Reconciliation in Cleveland, Ohio, was indicted by the commonwealth of Massachusetts on a charge of having aided and abetted a woman who obtained an illegal abortion in that state. Bob Hare had indeed counseled and referred a young woman to a doctor in Massachusetts. She drove from Cleveland to the doctor's office, was aborted, and was on her way home when she started experiencing severe cramping. Alarmed, she pulled off the highway and drove toward the first building she saw to seek assistance. In one of those strange quirks of fate, the building happened to be the headquarters of the highway patrol. Before providing her with medical assistance, the police demanded that she tell them what had happened; she did, including the names of both doctor and minister.

The commonwealth of Massachusetts, not known for its libertarian ways, proceeded to indict both doctor and minister. The doctor was able to retain one of the finest civil liberties lawyers in Massachusetts. A committee to raise funds for Bob Hare's defense was established immediately, and the support of Clergy Services around the country was enlisted. Fortunately the case against Bob Hare was never brought to trial, setting a precedent which would later be repeated.

The only other major challenge to clergy counselors occurred early in 1970 when a member of the Illinois CCS, Rabbi Max Ticktin, after referring a woman to a doctor in Detroit, was charged by the state of Michigan with conspiracy to commit abortion. This doctor had been under surveillance for some time, and it is possible that the involvement of the Illinois CCS in this case was purely coincidental. After a period of anxiety it became clear that no prosecution would ensue, and we attribute this to the excellent work of Spencer Parsons, chairman and spokesman for the Chicago CCS, whose public statements undoubtedly increased the reluctance of the authorities to engage in open warfare with the church.

None of the other challenges by law enforcement were nationally as threatening although there were local problems around the country which certainly alarmed counselors in that area. In New York, for example, we were called to testify at a grand jury hearing in the Bronx, which followed the uncovering of an "abortion ring" that had functioned for several years. This was the first and only time any legal agency indicated even moderate interest in our existence. True to our policy of referring to physicians practicing outside New York, we had no relationship with these abortionists. However, several Clergy Services in bordering states had been referring women to them as had two ex-members of the New York CCS. We assumed the district attorney's office had heard of clergy involvement and on that basis had subpoenaed us to testify.

Initially upset and fearful, we considered closing the New York CCS until after the grand jury had heard our testimony, but Ephraim London, our ever-calm and supportive attorney, advised us against taking what we thought would be a precautionary measure. He believed and succeeded in persuading us that to close down the CCS could be construed both as an admission of guilt in the Bronx case, and, in a larger sense, an acknowledgment that our counseling and referring of women for abortions was illegal, an admission we never made during those years.

While it probably helped to reinforce our cautious and conservative image, we chose to follow our lawyer's advice by agreeing to testify with complete openness about the New York CCS. Since others who had been subpoenaed had talked informally about refusing to cooperate and if necessary going to jail, they surely must have considered us cowards for refusing to join in the proposed martyrdom. Nevertheless, we consciously felt that it was important to avoid a confrontation in which we had no direct involvement and by staying out of jail continue to assist women.

Once again our fears were unwarranted. All the grand jury wanted to know was whether the New York CCS was "officially" involved with the doctors and whether we were profiting financially or receiving any kickbacks from abortionists in general. Our answer to both questions was no.

From then on, contact with the authorities came only at our request. In April, 1969, the New York CCS received a blackmail threat from a man claiming that his girl friend had obtained an abortion with our assistance; he warned that unless he was paid $5,000 within twenty-four hours, an official complaint would be registered against us with the New York City District Attorney's office. Advised that the CCS was a shoestring operation with limited funds, the blackmailer insisted that we get the money "from the doctors." He threatened to play "Russian Roulette" to see which of them would be exposed to the authorities if we refused to cooperate.

Unable to determine whether the blackmailer's girl friend had gone through the CCS and was actually in a position to identify and place in jeopardy any of our doctors, we agreed to cooperate with him. On the advice of our attorney, Ephraim London, we also informed the district attorney's office of the threat. They responded immediately, sending several detectives from the Racket Squad down to Judson Church. At their suggestion, we made arrangements to meet the blackmailer and deliver the money just across the street from the church. In true Grade B movie style, children's play money was purchased at the five and dime and dutifully wrapped in plain brown paper. Moody was wired for sound by the Racket Squad so that his conversation with the blackmailer could be monitored by detectives hidden in the church while the exchange was in progress. Before giving the payoff to the blackmailer, Moody asked what assurance he would have that another $5,000 would not be demanded sometime in the future. The blackmailer's response was that he was leaving the country and we would not be bothered again. Moody then handed over the package, at which point the Racket Squad moved in and arrested him with "the goods" in hand.

This experience confirmed our belief that observing the minimal legal strictures laid down by our attorney not only protected the CCS from harassment by the authorities but also entitled us to their protection. That incident ended on a sad note when we discovered that the "blackmailer" was the troubled nephew of a prominent Christian pastor and was wanted on a drug charge in California. After talks with his girl friend and visits with the young man in prison, we dropped charges and he was extradited to California to stand trial.

Months before the New York State abortion law was repealed, Aryeh Neier, then Executive Director of the New York Civil Liberties Union, was guest speaker at a gathering of New York Chiefs of Police. In response to a question about what he would do differently if he were the Police Commissioner of New York City, Neier stated that he would begin by eliminating all arrests then being made for "victimless crimes," such as prostitution, homosexuality, and abortion. When he finished, one police chief volunteered that they were doing just that with the Clergy Consultation Service on Abortion. From then on we knew we were home free.

For a brief time in 1969 we believed perhaps mistakenly that the federal government was investigating us. Our fear resulted from a visit by the Internal Revenue Service to the then coordinator of the New Jersey CCS, Charles Straut, Jr., seeking his cooperation in apprehending abortionists who had not paid taxes on their illicit incomes. The I.R.S. wanted the CCS to provide them with the names of such physicians. However, since the attitude of the CCS in principle toward abortionists was that they were fulfilling the highest calling of their profession, Straut did not offer aid. Shortly thereafter nearly a dozen abortionists around the country were arrested; we concluded that there was some connection between those arrests and the sudden interest of the I.R.S., but we were never able to establish that fact with certainty.

Although it took some time for the Clergy Services both individually and collectively to recognize the fact, we were developing strength which enabled us to negotiate with the doctors for both better service and lower costs to patients. In our infancy we simply accepted the price established by abortionists, never seriously questioning fairness. But within six months after the New York CCS opened, we had received many telephone solicitations and unscheduled visits from middlemen representing practicing abortionists. The solicitations usually followed the same scenario. We were told about some incredibly humane doctor who had decided to do abortions because his wife, or daughter, or sister, had been maimed or killed at the hands of an untrained, nonmedical practitioner. This personal tragedy had so changed the doctor's life that in complete disregard of his own safety and risking censure by professional colleagues, he had decided to offer his technical skills to womankind for a mere $600 per abortion. The middleman's function was to whet our interest in collaborating with this humanitarian by referring patients. In exchange we were generally offered a fifty-dollar kickback per patient "for the church." Oddly enough when we explained that we would not accept any financial remuneration but would be happy if the fee charged to women was lowered by fifty dollars, the response was negative. While middlemen would offer to set the money aside to cover abortions for indigent women whom we might refer, they were adamant about protecting and maintaining the existing price structure.

We see evidence that this trait has been carried over into the legal abortion market in New York City where certain facilities will routinely charge $25 or $50 less to patients referred by certain agencies who have arranged for a lower fee. Thus their top and public price, say $150, remains the same, and women aborted for $100 or $125 will refer a number of acquaintances over a period of time. These acquaintances have to pay the full fee of $150 because they were not "referred" by the proper agency. Such arrangements may have short-term advantages for the referral agency and *some* women, but by the same token it delays the agency's coming to grips with the problem of an inflated price structure which affects *all* people.

The middlemen we met were a breed unto themselves. Although they probably were well paid, we will never know if they fully understood the risks they were taking. The doctors whose services they were marketing functioned under pseudonyms and worked out of multiple offices, making it difficult for the authorities to catch up with them. Middlemen, on the other hand, were by the nature of their role fairly stable and consequently in greater jeopardy of being endangered by any irate woman whose abortion turned out badly.

With one or two exceptions, the middlemen were uneducated and seemed deficient in native intelligence. Those who visited us appeared to be laborers. They shared a naïveté about our purposes, goals, and concerns, which was reflected in the kickbacks they offered; it took some time to persuade them that "no" really meant "no."

One of our favorites was from New Jersey, and he stopped by Judson Church for well over six months before taking our lack of interest seriously. A rough looking but gentle man who worked in the construction industry, he generously offered to bring us building materials which the church might need instead of giving a dollar kickback. Since one of Judson's ongoing programs was the Judson Poets' Theater, the offer of materials which might be needed for set building, although tempting, was rejected. Months after, in what appeared to be perfect innocence, he offered to place a volunteer in the church office, and he gave the impression that he was truly hurt by our unwillingness to welcome this much needed assistance. Possibly our middleman friend had no hidden motives, but we reacted as though he did, and we never saw or heard from him again.

Though the solicitations increased (continuing even today), during the so-called "illegal days" we never referred any woman to an abortionist who had sought our "business." Perhaps it was nothing more than coincidence, but over the years we worked only with people whom we had sought out and with whom we had a very businesslike relationship, and none of *them* ever offered us anything in exchange. A well-known Michigan abortionist traveled to New York with his nurse/wife to solicit our referrals. Although he was impressive and had excellent credentials, we decided not to pursue a working relationship after he made it clear that he would terminate pregnancies beyond twelve weeks in an office setting despite our insistence that such procedures could endanger patients. Arrogance and a conviction of his superior skills made him willing to perform abortions up to twenty weeks under very minimal conditions, but we wanted no part in such risky practices. Some months later we received in the mail a bank draft for $1,000 accompanied by a note from the doctor stating that it was a contribution toward the work of the CCS. The doctor probably assumed that we would refer patients to him once we realized how profitable it could be. He must have been chagrined when we returned the check, for we never heard from him again.

Because we were puzzled by the solicitations of middlemen, one day out of curiosity we sat down and figured out that we were conducting a multimillion dollar business. The New York CCS was seeing ten thousand women a year, each of whom was paying approximately $600 for an abortion, and the role of the CCS was determining into whose pockets that $6,000,000 a year wound up. As the economic implications of our work became clear, we gradually began pressuring doctors to whom we referred patients to lower their fees and found them by and large perfectly willing to go along with our request. The advantages of regularly receiving well-screened referrals with no strings attached must have outweighed the financial loss to them.

If we found one of our doctors reluctant to go along with a reduction, we did not hesitate to threaten him with a loss of referrals. Since he was generally persuaded of our intentions, the price would be dropped. When one of our Puerto Rican doctors flatly refused to lower his fee, we had to follow through with our threat and simply channeled our counselees elsewhere for several weeks until he called and said he had changed his mind. Probably he was just testing to see if we meant what we said. Had we continued to refer patients after his refusal, it is unlikely that his price would have dropped.

As the Clergy Services expanded, particularly in the East, we sometimes found ourselves referring to the same abortionist who would charge a different price to Services in different states. Situations like this would occur when a particular CCS did not clear the doctor under consideration through National CCS before working out a referral arrangement. With some Services better at negotiating lower fees than others, there might be a discrepancy of $50 or $100 between what a Pennsylvania woman and a Massachusetts woman paid the same physician. The abortionists would rarely, if ever, let one CCS group know that he was also working with another CCS group, placing the burden of discovery on the clergy. Whenever we discovered such inequitable arrangements, we told the doctor that the fee to *all* Clergy Services would have to be the same or he would receive no referrals from any of us.

It would be misleading to assume that the wheeling and dealing with doctors was an automatic skill understood and shared equally by all Clergy Services. Sometimes when one CCS was attempting to negotiate a lower fee with a doctor whose referrals came from several Services, the negotiating Service had difficulty persuading the others that $550 was really too high a price for women to pay. Slowly and with real difficulty the clergy developed the sophistication which enabled them to see quite clearly that no matter how nice, an abortionist charging $600 or $500 or $400 per patient was still exploiting, and part of the role they needed to play with increasing frequency was that of consumer advocate.

The educational process was accelerated to some extent by an awareness that most women being served by the CCS were white and middle class. Very few low-income and ghetto women were seen by the clergy in the illegal days because it did not take long for the word to spread that the clergy could only help you if you had $500 or $600 plus travel expenses. Very few poor women could raise that kind of money, and consequently they continued to turn to midwives where possible, or in desperation they resorted to self-induced methods, which sometimes killed them. The Clergy Services, in the early days, had nothing to offer these women.

When the New York CCS examined its statistics after the first year and realized that virtually no black or Puerto Rican women were seeking our help, we concluded that we were doing something wrong—allowing the cost of an illegal abortion to remain prohibitively high. Each Clergy Service would eventually realize that in order to serve *all* women who were seeking abortions some effort would have to be made to lower the price. As that realization occurred, cooperation between local Services increased.

The change in England's abortion law provided most Clergy Services with an opportunity to negotiate for lower fees with homegrown abortionists. During the 1967–1968 period, not only were Clergy Services, wherever they existed, catering to a largely white, middle-class clientele, but we were providing assistance only for women whose pregnancies were less than twelve weeks along. After the first trimester, the only option then available was Japan, where the cost was prohibitively high ($2,000 including air fare).

Then, in April, 1968, Great Britain's Abortion Act went into effect, and London became a realistic alternative for many women with advanced pregnancies. While most found it impossible to raise $2,000 for Tokyo, many Americans were able to pull enough together to go to London. A woman eighteen weeks along needed roughly $1,000 for London. A woman with an early pregnancy needed only $800. In only a short time we saw that given a choice between an *illegal* abortion (costing $600) in Puerto Rico and a legal abortion (costing $800) in London, many women would choose the legal route despite the additional expense. The psychological and medical advantages of a legal termination were clearly worthwhile, and Clergy Services used this experience as a wedge with local practitioners who refused to drop their prices as long as there was no competition. They quickly changed their attitudes when they learned that we were sending to London women who normally would have been their patients.

Although we had followed newspaper reports of the changing British situation, we waited several months after the law went into effect before referring women to England. The delay was caused by our curiosity about the implementation of the new law, i.e., how and where abortions would be performed, what the costs would be, and whether foreigners would be welcome. Another cause for delay was the fact that we could not afford to send someone to London to check out the situation firsthand, a process which had always been a prerequisite for referral.

During May we were visited by several women in the Greenwich Village community who had traveled on their own to England, sought out doctors, and obtained abortions. After eliciting very thorough accounts of their experiences, we decided that in a "legal" situation perhaps it was not absolutely crucial to send our own observer. We began cautiously to refer women and requested that they make a follow-up, debriefing visit on their return. By July, 1970, when the New York abortion law was repealed, Clergy Services around the country were referring most of their advanced cases exclusively to one London doctor, David Sopher, a very gentle man, who served our women well. We began referral to Dr. Sopher on the basis of a report from a woman who had been aborted by another English physician. Following the procedure, she remained at the nursing home for some hours until released by the matron, never again seeing her doctor after the operation. Resting in bed, she observed that women who had been operated on by another doctor were being examined and discharged by their physician, and she was slightly envious of the personal care they were receiving. She learned the other doctor's name, and our initial contact with Dr. Sopher was made on the basis of her recommendation. After a short time the Clergy Services settled on Dr. Sopher as our primary British doctor.

The intervening years provided us with a great deal of experience and knowledge about what happens when a previously illegal act is made legal; much of this helped in anticipating and preparing for the change in New York's law. Solicitation, for example, was something we never expected would occur. We were somewhat stunned by the first visit from a fastidiously dressed British doctor who was touring the United States to meet with all potential referral sources. He was followed by other smooth-talking, well-educated, highly qualified English gynecologists who saw legal abortion as a golden opportunity. The belief that changing laws modified behavior was immediately shattered by the appearance of English entrepreneurs.

Consequently we were not too surprised when visiting medical solicitors cast doubt on Dr. Sopher's ability or when other London abortionists wrote and told us that they *used* to be in practice with him but were now striking out on their own and would like some of our referrals. There is probably not another area of medicine where doctors have felt so free to criticize their colleagues.

Since our women had always been hijacked by cab drivers in Puerto Rico, it was no great shock when London drivers followed suit. We had to warn women in the counseling session against believing any cab driver who claimed that Dr. Sopher was on vacation, arrested, or dead. Human nature is pretty much the same around the globe.

A year after the English law changed, we finally were able to visit England and get a firsthand impression of how that law was functioning for English women as well as foreigners. The visit was precipitated in part by the death of a young woman from Cleveland who had been referred by the Clergy Service to a rarely used London doctor. The autopsy report indicated that anesthesia was responsible, and indications of negligence on the part of the anesthesiologist resulted in added pressure for us to make an early visit. The report of this visit was prepared for all Clergy Services (then operating in ten states), and it pointed up some of the problems we would later have to confront on our own soil.

While we knew that under National Health Service the British receive free medical treatment, we didn't know that they can only apply for treatment at a hospital in their own residential district. The consequences of this residency requirement are obvious. While many hospitals in London regularly perform abortions without any hassle at all (one National Health Service doctor we spoke to does six a day), the situation throughout the rest of the Commonwealth is less encouraging. Reports have it that no doctors or hospitals in the Midlands, for example, perform abortions under any circumstances. Since women residing outside of London are ineligible in NHS hospitals in London, they are flocking there anyway seeking to make arrangements at private nursing homes. (There is a regular Friday night train from Birmingham to London for this purpose—arrangements having been made in advance with a private physician.)

In London there are roughly seven nursing homes licensed to do abortions. They are owned and operated by businessmen/doctors who hire nursing staff and equip the home with operating theater, medications, etc. The owners then rent beds and nursing care to physicians who pay $100 per day per patient for use of the home's facilities. Medical standards for the homes are set by the government; they are not observed by the owners, however.

Based on observations at the homes we visited, the government's standards are often sacrificed to the owner's desire to keep the beds filled. At one home we were told by the Matron that there were times when the bed linen was changed three times a day (each change representing a different patient).

After the death of the Cleveland girl, the government started investigating the nursing homes and found, for example, that blood which might be necessary in an emergency was not kept available. The government gave the homes 30 days to correct certain flagrant violations, but the feeling is that the owners will do only the minimum required to avoid losing their licenses.

Because the homes are privately owned, the doctors are completely dependent on the owner's goodwill for regular use of space. This puts them in a poor bargaining position when it comes to improving, particularly, the post-operative care received by their patients. The law requires that a woman who has undergone an abortion remain in the hospital for a minimum of 24 hours afterwards. Few women are kept that long, and were the doctors to protest they would be blacklisted by the nursing home owners. The owners (also in violation of the law) admit patients to the home and then insist that one of the doctors working there operate. Despite the illegality of this situation the doctors have no choice but to cooperate.

The report went on to evaluate several English doctors, including the one who had operated on the Cleveland woman, and it concluded with a strong recommendation that Dr. Sopher was the only one about whom we could be completely confident.

> Sopher is a warm and gentle man and our patients seem to like and trust him (while the nursing home staff dislikes his care and caution in the operating room; one matron claimed that other doctors can terminate two pregnancies in the time it takes Sopher to do one; this means $200 to them instead of $100 for the same length of time). . . . We think the CCS is lucky to have Sopher's cooperation, that we can feel confident about him medically as well as ethically, and that we should continue our relationship with him.

Because of the system under which private abortions were performed and the relatively small number of patients we referred, we never succeeded in affecting the English price structure. The average fee for a first trimester abortion was about $300, although some physicians were charging as much as $750. With patients coming from all over Europe as well as the United States, there was no way to apply collective pressure for lower fees. However, what we learned during those few years guided our later efforts in New York to have all Clergy Services in the eastern United States refer to one abortion facility, thereby making it both responsible and responsive to our concerns for quality of care and costs.

While Clergy Services made far less of an impact on the English abortion scene than on illegal American abortionists, the experience gave us a preview of both the problems and possibilities that would await us in the future when the New York State law changed.

By July 1, 1970, affiliates of the National CCS were operating in twenty states, with the heaviest concentration in the East. We began to examine possible next steps in our struggle to open up to all women the right, and the means to implement that right, to decide about abortion.

The Making of a Model: A New Kind of Health Facility

The failure of the New York State Legislature to take any action on the abortion issue in 1969, combined with our growing security in relationship to the legal authorities, led us to look for a new and more dramatic way to challenge the abortion statute. The next logical and meaningful step seemed clear: open an abortion facility in New York City in violation of the law. Our two parallel goals would be to demonstrate the feasibility and safety of performing abortions prior to ten weeks of gestation as an outpatient, ambulatory office procedure; and second, to expose the hypocrisy of a law which allowed "therapeutic" abortions for the rich but denied them to the poor. In order to fulfill these goals, we would follow, and in a very real sense mock, the prohibitively expensive hospital procedures.

The year before we had fantasized about setting up an "abortion ship" just outside the three-mile limit under a foreign (Japanese) flag. We even went so far as to have a friend whose specialty was maritime law investigate the implications of such a project. Concluding that there was some risk involved, he recommended that we attempt to implement the idea. He foresaw only one real danger: the support of the country under whose flag our ship sailed might collapse should the U.S. government bring pressure to bear. We halfheartedly and unsuccessfully tried to raise funds for the ship, all the while envisioning a steady stream of women descending on New York's Hudson River with oars slung over their shoulders, ready to row out to the ship. The philanthropic reaction was negative. Then when our medical advisors raised doubts about safety, the plan was permanently filed away.

With the unanimous consent of members of the New York

CCS, we held exploratory meetings with Aryeh Neier of the N.Y.C.L.U. and our lawyer, Ephraim London. Perhaps because London had always insisted that we act in a circumspect if not cautious manner, we were astonished and totally unprepared for his enthusiastic reaction. London and Neier both believed that while the legal risks of establishing a clinic were greater than those we faced in the early days of the New York CCS, we might, by acting judiciously, "get away with it." Basically, "acting judiciously" meant that no one would profit financially from the clinic, and everything about it would be open and above board.

With the backing of London and Neier, we began seeking friendly gynecologists and psychiatrists who would be willing, perhaps, to risk their careers by joining us in this venture. While several gynecologists responded affirmatively and met with us over a period of months, only one, Dr. Bernard Nathanson, was absolutely committed. Nathanson had helped pioneer a liberal interpretation of the restrictive New York abortion law at St. Luke's Hospital. Through his efforts and with his assistance we had been able to obtain therapeutic abortions for minors, married women, and some poor women, none of whom really qualified under a strict definition of the law. Each legal abortion we helped arrange at St. Luke's and elsewhere—always more complicated because of the psychiatric consent necessary—was an occasion for celebration. It seemed reasonable that the more therapeutic abortions were done, the more commonplace the procedure would become, particularly for the medical personnel. Also attitudes would be changed by firsthand contact with the patients, and in the long run the legislative picture would be affected. While Nathanson was not the only gynecologist to push his hospital to do more, he was one of the few advocates of abortion law reform who was also willing to practice what he preached. To our disappointment we were able to find only one sympathetic psychiatrist, and even he wavered as time passed. This hesitation was perhaps because our plans called for psychiatrists simply to provide "rubber stamp" approval to a woman's request for an abortion, not a terribly attractive role for a professional.

By December, 1969, we had drawn up a confidential prospectus for a Reproduction Crisis Facility under the auspices of the New York Clergy Consultation Service on Abortion. Its stated purposes were:

1. To establish a pilot project which would seek to prove the feasibility and safety of performing abortions prior to ten weeks in an outpatient, ambulatory, office procedure.

2. To assist women with problem pregnancies by providing counseling, examinations, psychiatric consultations, medical assistance, and contraceptive education.

3. To provide women with safe, inexpensive, and humane treatment regardless of ability to pay.

The concerns of London and Neier were clearly incorporated into the prospectus:

It is a significant purpose of the experimental project to establish the feasibility of providing medical services to women with problem pregnancies at a minimum cost without refusing service to anyone because she lacks funds. The facility will be a completely nonprofit operation.

All personnel (except unpaid clergy counselors) would receive salaries commensurate with going rates for professionals in the medical field.

A C.P.A. would be hired to handle all bookkeeping and checkwriting work. The accountant would make quarterly reports which could be (if necessary) open to the public at any time.

The New York State law in 1969 required that a woman obtain letters from two psychiatrists attesting that her life would be in jeopardy if the pregnancy were carried to term. These letters were then presented to the Committee on Therapeutic Abortions of her gynecologist's hospital. If the committee approved, the abortion could be performed. If it disapproved, she was denied the abortion no matter how compelling her reasons might be. Since most hospitals had fixed quotas for therapeutic abortions (none wanted to become known as abortion mills), applying for one often resembled Russian Roulette.

In the facility we planned, a woman would also require two psychiatric recommendations. We intended, however, to locate psychiatrists who believed that *any* woman contemplating an *illegal* abortion was a threat to her own life and thus eligible for a therapeutic abortion. Our Committee on Therapeutic Abortions would be composed of prominent medical and lay professionals who would, without question, accept the psychiatrists' recommendations. Consequently no woman medically eligible for a first trimester ambulatory abortion would be refused service at our clinic.

The real difference between our administrative procedures and those of New York hospitals would be the elimination of red tape and substantial reduction in the expense. Since the New York law did not specifically require that abortions be performed in hospitals (that practice was dictated by medical tradition), the authorities would be hard pressed for legal grounds upon which to deny us the right to exist.

After some months of holding small, private meetings at Judson Church, the participants decided to bring together several key people in the abortion movement for the purpose of informing them and eliciting their support for our project. Included in that larger group were luminaries like Dr. Alan Guttmacher, Dr. Robert Hall, and Harriet Pilpel, Esq. After a few gatherings it became clear that support from them would be delayed. As one participant wrote, "I do not think we are ready to act upon it." Several proposed that discussions continue for an indefinite period until there was unanimous agreement upon every point.

Foolish though it may have seemed, our nucleus group decided to go ahead without the support of the more cautious. They could continue to meet and discuss, but the women who needed abortions might not be able to wait until a "perfect" plan was developed. Following the experience of the New York CCS, we were prepared to strike out with an imperfect effort that would in time be modified and/or improved. At the very least, women would be receiving abortion services which were superior in every way to those offered by "illegal" abortionists.

As we began to develop plans for the project, we determined that 2,300 square feet would be needed. Everyone agreed that the clinic should be located close to Judson Church since it would be operating under the auspices of the New York CCS, and Arthur Levin, a friend of Judson, began scouting the area. Nathanson began preparing a list of equipment needed to outfit the clinic, some of which would be purchased outright and some of which would be rented. Faced with the prospect of being closed down by the authorities, we did not want to invest too much money in medical equipment.

Our first obstacle centered around the rental of office space. Signing a lease for one or two years would legally commit us to paying rent whether or not we were forcibly constrained from operating, and it was a foregone conclusion that structural changes would need to be made in any rented space, an expensive necessity that could conceivably be wasted. In the absence of legal guarantees that we would not be challenged by the authorities, we had no choice but to proceed on the assumption that our clinic would indeed be shut down. Such a presupposition forced us to avoid any long-term lease arrangements or investments in structural changes for a facility we might use only briefly.

The initial money required to get the clinic going was estimated at $40,000. While a foundation grant was hoped for, a loan was a more realistic possibility. The commitment to repay either a foundation or a bank discouraged us from any long-term rental. In our preliminary budget we had estimated income at roughly $5,000 per week and expenses at about $3,000 per week. On that basis if all went well and we were permitted to remain open for five months, the $40,000 could be repaid. If we continued beyond five months, our estimated surplus would be over $60,000 in the first year. This surplus was to be plowed back into improved and expanded patient services, lowered fees, and, if necessary, charitable contributions, so that at the end of a year an official audit would show no profit whatsoever. This was consistent with our own philosophy as well as our lawyers' recommendations.

Sometime in January or February of 1970, it appeared certain that physical space for the clinic could not be obtained unless we were willing to sign a one-year lease. Coincidentally, a brownstone owned by and located behind Judson Church, which for two years had housed a residence for runaway youth, was vacated as that experimental program ended. Through the years the brownstone, a three-story structure, had housed the Judson Health Center and had been a residence for artists and writers in training, as well as the residence of the associate minister and church custodian. In the absence of church plans for other programs to occupy that space, it was inevitable that the question of its availability for the abortion clinic would arise. Faced with no other alternative and determined to carry through with this extended testing of the New York law, we eventually asked Judson to house the abortion facility.

The Judson Church Board Minutes of March 24, 1970, read as follows:

> The Board considered a proposal from Howard Moody that the second floor of (Judson) House be renovated for use as an "abortorium." Howard

explained that whether or not the abortion repeal bill is passed, a model will be needed to show women, doctors and hospitals that abortions can be safely performed under office conditions. Setting up such a program would probably cost about $40,000, and there should be little difficulty about raising this. The volume (of patients) would start at about 35 per week and would hopefully increase with the recruiting of additional doctors. Cost of the operation should average about $75 with patients paying according to their resources. Ron Bailey reported that the (Judson) House Committee had approved the proposal. . . . The Board voted to accept the recommendation of the (Judson) House Committee giving authority to the staff to move ahead. . . .

In the three years that Judson had housed and given staff to the New York CCS, the church's own commitment to the needs and rights of women had been strengthened. Like the clergy counselors it was willing to risk testing the law on new and potentially more dangerous ground.

Early in April, 1970, the New York State Legislature unexpectedly, by a margin of one vote, passed the Cooke/Leichter Abortion Reform bill. Within days we received a call from Dr. Hale Harvey in another state, asking if we would like him to come to New York and set up a clinic which would be ready to open on July 1, the day New York's abortion law would go into effect. Our answer was an enthusiastic yes. Harvey's offer to come to New York made it unnecessary for the CCS to establish a model abortion facility; we were confident that Dr. Harvey would do it instead.

To explain this decision to let Dr. Harvey establish the clinic rather than ourselves, it is necessary to backtrack just a bit. Early in 1969 we had been visited by a young woman just returned from a year in London where she had done research on sex education and abortion referral groups. She thought that we would be interested in learning more about the English situation. Born in Oklahoma, schooled in New Orleans, she planned to enter the graduate program in philosophy at New York University. At this initial meeting with Barbara Pyle, then twenty-two years old, we heard for the first time about her friend Hale Harvey III. Dr. Harvey had practiced medicine in the South, and taught philosophy and ethics in a university, and in 1969 was devoting his energies to epidemiological research in medicine and public health. His area of interest and the subject of his doctoral thesis was "An Epidemiological Approach Toward Making Good Decisions About Ethical Problems in Medicine and Public Health," with special emphasis on sexuality. Deeming abortion an epidemic, Harvey had set his own ethical path: He would perform abortions despite the illegality of the procedure in his state. Our interest was more than mildly aroused by this meeting, and Barbara Pyle left with a promise to invite Dr. Harvey to visit with us to discuss his future plans and explore possible areas of cooperation.

The meeting with Dr. Harvey took place some weeks later, and it was the only time we ever invited an abortionist to meet with us at Judson. Harvey turned out to be a curiously impersonal but totally dedicated man. After explaining his theory of abortion as an epidemic (we already knew that he was absolutely correct about this) and describing the process which had led him to decide to perform abortions, Harvey concluded by offering his services to us. Impressed by his sincerity, we forced ourselves to beware that beneath a surface of concern and conviction, hidden from view, must lie some form of self-interest. But during the year that we referred patients to him, we never detected any secret motive, only genuine compassion and concern for the welfare of women.

With our expression of interest at that time, Harvey returned home and opened a suite of offices in a downtown hotel. Referral arrangements were worked out; and at Harvey's insistence the fee which patients paid was to be determined by the clergy counselor at $100, $200, or $300. At no time during the year which followed did Harvey ever complain or indicate that we were setting fees too low.

Through that experience we learned what a difference it made to patients when they felt the doctor had a genuine interest in their well-being. Harvey had a unique style and used his imagination to provide extras that no other "illegal" abortionist would have even considered. For example, he put colorful potholders on the stirrups of the operating table for both the comfort and pleasure of patients; he told patients calling for appointments to bring along their knitting or magazines or something else to occupy them while waiting; he had cokes and cookies available postoperatively for patients who had not eaten for twelve hours; and he mimeographed a sheet of things to do for patients with free time before catching their return flight. This combination of extras, plus excellent medical skill, made women feel good about the doctor, themselves, and the experience. Patients back from their appointments repeatedly told us that they had been "treated like an individual," and we understood how important that was. With the passage of time the consistently good reports brought back by women we had referred persuaded us that Dr. Harvey was basically sincere.

With this experience behind us it seemed too good to be true when Hale Harvey telephoned in April, 1970, to discuss his plans for establishing a clinic in New York City. We believed that any facility which he designed would include in its structure the concerns we shared in common: low cost, quality care, humane treatment, and a willingness to serve the poor. On that score we were not disappointed. The nonprofit facility that Harvey founded, the Center for Reproductive and Sexual Health, is a tribute to his deep concern for the abortion problem and its humane treatment.

Dr. Harvey had established the clinic which we expected would be the model clinic that we believed was needed. But there were still many problems to come. It is doubtful that there had ever been in the annals of social change and legal reform such a dramatic victory as we experienced in New York State with the repeal of the eighty-three-year-old abortion law. A testimony to that fact is how ill-prepared all concerned were for the problems which were to come. Perhaps the Clergy Consultation Service was better prepared than most groups and institutions simply because the firsthand experience both with referral and medical practices including the medical economics of abortion forearmed us for the ensuing contests.

Our task until this point had been primarily pastoral, using our offices as concerned professionals in counseling women and acting as enablers in discovering and maintaining safe, efficient medical sources for procurement of an abortion. With the changing of the law so that abortion up to the twenty-fourth week was permissible, the task of the clergy shifted from the pastoral to the prophetic. Now anyone who knows anything about the history of church/world relations knows that pastors are indulged but prophets are stoned. In our new role the CCS in New York had to insure on behalf of the rest of the country the kind of medical delivery system that would afford lowest-cost, quality abortions for the thousands of women who would begin seeking care in a place where the procedure was now legal. The challenge before us was fairly clear. How could we utilize and capitalize upon the vast experience we had garnered in the three years of "illegal" counseling and referral of women and the identification of competent medical resources? We had developed over the years several firm convictions about the innovations that would be necessary to provide safe, low-cost, and humane abortions in the city when the law changed.

The first and most significant conviction we held, one which went against all medical opinion with the exception of that of a few doctors who had experience with outpatient abortions, was that first trimester abortions (first twelve weeks) need not medically, and for economy should not, be performed in regular hospital settings, but rather they should be performed in ambulatory, outpatient facilities (known in the trade as "free-standing clinics"). Our adversaries were the Department of Health, Health and Hospitals Corporation, and most of the medical profession, including ardent abortion law reformers like Dr. Robert Hall. As far as those people were concerned, the CCS was a group of nonprofessional, inexperienced laymen. After all, what did a group of clergy know about medical matters? This prejudice on the part of the physicians was understandable, but it overlooked our heavy experience which had taught us a great deal about abortion practices and techniques. In three years CCS nationally had referred perhaps 100,000 women for office abortions without a single fatality.

In the four months between passage of the 1970 New York Abortion Law and July 1, its effective date, Hale Harvey and Barbara Pyle created the first freestanding abortion facility in the United States. The Center for Reproductive and Sexual Health (or "Women's Services," as the clinic came to be called), opened its doors on July 1 in a professional medical building on East 73rd Street in Manhattan, innovating procedures that would later be duplicated elsewhere in New York as well as in other states.

Harvey relied heavily on his earlier experience. Unconsciously following Frank Lloyd Wright's architectural principle that "form follows function," he rejected the mythology of the traditional medical establishment, which would have dictated an impersonal and inhumane hospital atmosphere. He trusted instead in his own knowledge of what was desirable and necessary to insure patient safety; he built into that facility a component of compassion that was by itself revolutionary in the history of health care in this country. A suite of perhaps a dozen doctors' offices was rented, each with a tiny private waiting room. The offices, commonly referred to as procedure rooms, contained only an operating table, a vacuum aspirator, and small sterilizer—all designed to be nonthreatening to the patient, who in such a space could observe effortlessly everything that was happening.

The outer waiting rooms were converted into counseling offices where young women, many of whom had undergone abortions in Harvey's original office, would explain in detail, using a pelvic model for illustration, precisely what would occur when the patient entered the procedure room. The nurse/counselors had been hired for the facility on the basis of their empathy and sensitivity toward patients, a quality which Harvey considered to be more important than education and experience. The role of the nurse/counselor was to alleviate any fears and anxieties that the patient had about abortion while at the same time preparing her both psychologically and intellectually for the procedure.

To the early horror of the New York medical community, counselors, not all of whom were R.N.'s, assisted the doctor during the abortion. This practice enabled them to provide continuous reassurance and comfort to the patient, explaining each step along the way just before it happened and eliminating the patient's fear of the unexpected.

The facility was decorated in bright, cheerful colors in order to create a warm, intimate, and friendly atmosphere. Harvey's conviction was that even a healthy patient would feel sick, in the face of a cold, sterile hospital environment; since abortion was not a sickness, the atmosphere associated with hospitals needed to be avoided.

In its first month, some seven hundred women, all referred by Clergy Services in surrounding states, had abortions at Women's Services. Glowing reports began flowing in from patients who had returned home ecstatic about the humane and compassionate care they had received. It was immediately clear that Harvey and Pyle had created the ideal setting for the delivery of a new kind of health care, a fact which was not lost on the entrepreneurs, businessmen, and doctors who in the following months opened dozens of similar facilities around the city. Women's Services was the model they had to duplicate in order to arouse the interest of other referral groups. Copy and compete they did, even on fees, not voluntarily but only because the existence of Women's Services allowed them no choice.

The day before Women's Services opened, we went to see it for the first time with Harvey and Pyle. On the drive uptown, Harvey turned to us and asked how much patients should be charged for the procedure. Since the lowest cost for an abortion up to that time had been $300, we said, "Let's try $200." Without a moment's hesitation he said, "Fine, we'll start with that." He also suggested that Clergy Service counselors should, at their own discretion, be able to reduce the fee to $100 or even to nothing. In the belief that no woman should receive a free abortion, that both her dignity and self-respect would be damaged by such charity, we persuaded a very reluctant Harvey to agree that poor women would have to pay a token fee of $25. It seems incredible in retrospect that we (the clergy) had to *force* Harvey to agree to such an arrangement, but he had brought to New York the same air of innocence and compassion which had character-ized his practice earlier.

The task of the National Clergy Service, upon seeing the kind of facility that was developed in those early months, was to keep that clinic alive, with statistics showing its relatively low com-plication rate and with consistently favorable feedback from pa-tients who were referred by Clergy Consultation Services. In order to achieve this goal, we did two things. The first was to undertake a continuous monitoring of all its services to patients, passing along to the staff the benefit of our endless feedback. Two com-plaint forms were developed at the beginning. One was for clergy counselors to use in reporting any major or minor problem which they or their counselees had encountered at Women's Services. The other complaint form was used by nurse/counselors at Women's Services to provide clergy with reports of any striking weaknesses or omissions in their counseling. This two-way re-porting system, profitable to both Women's Services and the CCS, was most beneficial to the patient herself. We also did all we could to encourage licensing of the clinic, defending it before health and hospital officials, all of whom were suspicious of this fledgling upstart of a facility that within six months was doing as many first trimester abortions as all the municipal hospitals in New York City combined.

Our desire to develop a model health facility which would demonstrate that first trimester abortions could be done safely out of the hospital in an ambulatory, outpatient medical clinic with humane care at a low cost would have been a fantasy had we not possessed a national referral network. This network proved to be a resource much more important than money. For some three years the network had been consistently concerned about supplying safe and, wherever possible, low-cost abortions to women in a high-demand/low-supply black market situation.

The existence of this network composed of clergy and lay people across the country who cared and were committed to working together in the creation of a highly professional, effective, voluntary referral service was what made possible the origin and development of Women's Services. It was literally the clinic the clergy built, not without the medical creativity and administrative know-how of its founders Harvey and Pyle, but certainly the clergy were the decisive factor in its evolution. The volume of women coming from Clergy Services, the strong sense of patient advocacy, the follow-up and feedback of the clergy— all enabled us to exert significant formative influence on Women's Services.

Let's look at the record of what the cooperative action of the Clergy Services accomplished in the area of price control during the first two years of that facility. CCS had long experience with the problem of price while dealing with "illegal" abortionists in the days before liberalized laws. CCS had set the price at the opening of Women's Services in July, 1970, at $200 (that was the lowest going rate that we knew). With the help of a large, steady volume of patients, that price was pushed down to $125 within one year. Let it be understood that in New York City during the same period, an abortion in a doctor's office (first trimester) was, and still is, $300, and hospital abortions ranged from $300 to $500. Since WS was one of the first clinics to be licensed by the N.Y. State Department of Health and approved by the N.Y.C. Health Department, it was natural that most abortion clinics would look at this facility and imitate its best features. Some of the commercial clinics voluntarily did so, but others only involuntarily lowered their prices in order to compete with WS.

The establishment of a reasonable fee for first trimester abortions in New York City was singularly due to the cooperative venture of CCS and WS.

Further, the CCS effected through the creation of WS not only the lowest priced abortion in the whole country (California was still locked into the hospital system), but it also helped to build into the facility's structure consistent, concrete financial aid to the poor and the young who could not afford the full fee. Women's Services and its Board of Trustees accepted a formula to be applied nationally with Clergy Services and later with other groups that wanted to refer patients: one out of every four patients referred could pay only the token fee of $25. The national formula was very important because women in surrounding states closest to New York City, even though they were poor, could be referred in larger numbers so long as the national percentage of patients paying $25 did not exceed 25 percent of the total patient load. For example, at times New Jersey CCS would refer two out of every four women at the token fee, but the Iowa CCS would refer only one out of seven women at the rate of $25, thus providing the economic balance needed to meet the formula. It was amazing that this could be done by a clinic with the lowest top fee in New York.

However, this generosity on the part of WS initiated at the insistence of National CCS was later to prove the source of the clinic's most serious problems. When abortion procedures began being performed in large numbers by many doctors in many different facilities, referral groups sprang up all over the country. Some of these were commercial and others were nonprofit, including groups such as Planned Parenthood, Women's Liberation, and college counseling services. These groups developed their own relationships among the competing clinics in New York City with one omission: a hard-nosed deal that would include a formula for assisting the poor. Consequently, women who could pay were referred to one or another commercial clinic, and the poor were referred to the Clergy Services whose medical facility in New York took all the poor, as they had from the beginning. No group "dumped the poor" on WS with malice aforethought. They just did not understand the long-range implications of their actions, namely, that they would eventually scuttle the facility whose increasing ratio of service to the poor might unbalance its nonprofit economy. These referral groups suffered from a normal provincialism and failed to recognize that abortion is a national problem. Clergy Services understood that better and encouraged the national office to negotiate in their name because of the power of corporate action. This Nader-like principle is the secret at the heart of consumer advocacy. If a person only cares that *one* woman with a financial problem gets helped and has no perspective on *all* the women in the other parts of the country who have the same problem, what is forfeited is the united action that could make available a lot more help for many more women. If the white middle-class clergy or lay counselor in Kansas doesn't care whether the poor of Connecticut get abortions, then that counselor doesn't understand the difference it makes in regard to what clinic or under what terms referrals are made.

When the commercial clinics put their traveling sales or public relations people on the road to drum up business for their enterprises, they counted on the well-worn practice of divide and conquer as far as Clergy Services were concerned. They counted on gullibility and ignorance of the national picture on the part of new referral groups, or perhaps they counted on blowing a few egos with a lot of personal attention, phone calls, paid trips to New York, and the promise of taking care of your "poor people." This technique was especially effective west of Ohio, and it was particularly interesting that the soliciting agents of commercial clinics never tried to persuade Pennsylvania or New Jersey Clergy Services to refer their clients, including their "poor." Had they done so, they would have been forced to live up to their promises. The poor of Nebraska or Michigan can rarely raise the transportation money needed to get them to New York, a fact which the commercial clinics banked on.

Should Women's Services go under because it tries to serve the poor in large volume while referral and counseling groups, for various reasons, make individual arrangements with commercial clinics in New York, we will have lost a very important tool in implementing the repeal law so that abortions are made available to *all* women regardless of their ability to pay.

The fact that Women's Services is a nonprofit facility, whose application for tax-exemption is pending, distinguishes it from many clinics in New York to which women are being referred. The significance of this fact is clear: individual persons are not making huge profits from the clinic. Women's Services and the two Planned Parenthood clinics in New York City are the only nonprofit outpatient facilities serving the poor in any kind of volume. Of course this factor is no guarantee in and of itself that these institutions will have superior services; but it does mean that because no profits have to be made, no shortcuts have to be taken in medical care, no trimming of personnel to cut payroll, no shortchanging of service in behalf of "economy" to maintain profits. Whatever money Women's Services makes (after its $250,000 debt is paid) will be plowed back into patient care and structural improvements, as well as the further lowering of the $125 fee and the assisting of more poor. That distinction is the fundamental case to be made for the nonprofit facility as long as its services and care are of a high quality. After its tax-exemption is received, this clinic will eventually be able to apply for tax-deductible monies now available to private, voluntary hospitals that serve a community. We know of many community hospitals with great endowments and foundation help which have not served the indigent with anything like the faithfulness of Women's Services. Since July, 1970, Women's Services has performed medical procedures for over six thousand women at $25 or less. What other commercial clinic which boasts its humanitarian nature and willingness to accept patients at reduced fees can match that record?

Another innovation in health care which was built into the structure and functioning of Women's Services by the CCS is the role of "patient advocacy." During the first year after abortion became legal in New York, National CCS played that part in behalf of the Clergy Services. As we saw the growing need to have someone at the clinic whose primary task was the patient's care and liaison with the counselors who referred her, we prevailed upon the Board of Trustees of Women's Services to create such a position. Seeing the value of the proposal, the Board complied and Marchieta Ceppos was then employed by and is answerable only to the Board. Her major function is the care of the patient, not how much money the clinic can save, not the labor problems of workers in the clinic, not even the protection of medical and administrative personnel who goof off; her job is to see that the patient consistently gets what she paid for in both medical services and human warmth and concern. The welfare and financial stability of the clinic is secondary to the patient's needs. It would not be an overstatement to say that if there were such an ombudsman in every hospital and health facility in New York a revolution in health care might be possible. We know of no commercial abortion clinic which has or would institute that kind of self-critical watchdog of medical standards and patient care.

Finally, to insure the kind of high quality facility incorporating the concerns the Clergy Services have for patients they refer, Women's Services set up in its charter a Board of Trustees made up of unpaid, nonstaff, public spirited citizens whose only stake in that clinic is to ensure that it functions financially and medically so that it may continue to furnish low-cost, quality-care medical assistance to women in need of abortions.

Women's Services is the clinic that Clergy Services made happen, and without it abortion facilities in New York would be very different. The purpose and strategy that went into the creation of Women's Services with its unique structure is what sets it apart from and makes it different from any commercial clinic. If the advocacy of Clergy Services is to have any permanent meaning, it must be translated into support of a model that we hope will be duplicated in every state and region when the changes in the law occur. But Clergy Services across the country will not need any other first trimester facility as a standard for competitive pricing as long as patients are being referred to New York City. Were the Clergy Services to forsake this medical facility (with its capacity to treat one thousand patients each week) for matters of personal whim, or some small "convenience" or gimmick offered by its competitors, it would demonstrate its failure to grasp the long-range goal of real consumer advocacy in this new medical delivery system.

When the Changes Come: Implementing the Law

What proved to be a far-reaching initial decision, after the legislature acted, was that on July 1, 1970, when the new law went into effect, the Clergy Consultation Service in New York would dissolve. This decision, which later was to prove perhaps premature, was based on the premise that the decision about abortion really should be left between a woman and her doctor and that no person, either psychiatrist or clergy, should be involuntarily placed between a woman and her physician. There was a lot of talk in Albany that an amendment might be added to the law which would make it mandatory for a woman to see a social worker or professional of some kind before she could attain an abortion. We could see the possibility of clergy taking the place of psychiatrists as patsys for the Ob/Gyn profession again removing from the doctor responsibility for granting a woman, barring medical contraindication, this elective procedure. The proposed amendment never developed, but the possibility helped us decide to go out of business the day the law changed. For three years the clergy had been spending large amounts of their pastoral time counseling women; and they were tired, deserved to rest, and wanted to go back to other causes and responsibilities which they had neglected. All of us were ready to counsel any woman who wanted help in making her decision, and all the clergy agreed to stand ready for that possible need. But the ensuing months proved that most women do not require counseling once the stigma of involvement in an "illicit" act is removed and safe procedures are provided in hospitals and clinics. Of course women continue to worry or agonize over the decision, but in most cases they do not require the services of a professional when abortion has become a simple elective medical procedure.

The next important decision we made after disbanding the clergy as counselors was to reconstitute them as advocates of women seeking abortions in light of the guidelines of the Health Department and the conservative medical profession's insistence that abortions must be performed in hospitals. We felt that the hospital system in New York City, with a built-in prejudice against this new procedure and already overtaxed and understaffed, would create chaos in a new medical delivery system. We decided, therefore, that the clergy could become "watchdogs" of hospital abortions and advocates of women hassled and harassed by an unsympathetic hospital bureaucracy. We created for the purpose of accomplishing this task an organization called Clergy and Lay Advocates for Hospital Abortion Performance. It had a phone and a coordinator, Ms. Barbara Krassner, a member of Judson Church and a fervent women's rights' advocate. Any woman who had trouble getting an abortion in a New York City hospital could call the number and receive assistance for getting her abortion at the earliest date. When necessary we would intercede for her.

The reason for our work was not only to facilitate the woman's abortion but also to amass evidence of the inadequacy of the hospital system to absorb both first and second trimester abortions, as well as the economic infeasibility of such a system. On July 1, the day the law went into effect, all the bureaucrats of the medical establishment and the Health and Hospitals Corporation were assuring everyone that there was no need to talk about setting up freestanding clinics, that the hospitals of the city could easily do all the abortions required, and besides clinics were not all that safe. On that date the backlog of women already registered at hospitals and waiting for abortions was 717. On August 12, the backlog was 1380 women. On September 17, it was reported that the number of women waiting was 2500. At the rate of 100 abortions a day being performed in New York hospitals, that was a three-week waiting list. By September 18 when the Health and Hospitals Corporation claimed that the abortion program in city hospitals was a "success," the waiting period for women seeking merely to be examined averaged from three to four weeks in length. Women in the early stages of pregnancy began to be shuffled from one hospital to another, and cash in advance was being demanded of even the poor, despite the public posture of the Corporation that no resident of New York City would be denied a hospital abortion whether she could pay for it or not.

From July 1 to October 1 we gathered documentation on the whole hospital system and its failure to provide an efficient, safe, low-cost abortion for women requiring that service. We were able to substantiate our charge that only the law had changed. Most of the bad characteristics of the "illegal" days—the victimization, the cruelty to women—were still with us; only the characters of the problem had changed. Under the Health and Hospitals Corporation's implementation of the law, a woman could spend days and weeks being shoved from one hospital to the next before she found someone willing and able to help her. Often this meant that she was delayed from an early, safe, ambulatory abortion (performed until twelve weeks) to a difficult and sometimes traumatic saline abortion (performed after the sixteenth week of pregnancy), unnecessarily endangering her health. There was no referral system worthy of the name for pregnant women. Under the law, doctors (now called not "abortionists" but "Ob/Gyns") were charging the same prices as the old illegal abortionists. The poor and the young who had suffered the most when abortions were illegal were still having the hardest time.

The Health and Hospitals Corporation pretended that the system was performing beautifully and encouraged the Board of Health to pass stringent guidelines for freestanding clinics that made them mini-hospitals. The Board of Health's inclusion of these regulations in the Health Code was an ill-founded and precipitous decision, based on no pragmatic experience and made without proper evaluation of the hospital system's handling of the abortion demand in the city. The medical establishment failed to mobilize public and voluntary hospitals to provide sufficient abortion services, to establish any adequate city-wide referral system, or to investigate means of terminating early pregnancies in alternative medical facilities. This failure added up to a nonfulfillment of their promise to provide the women of New York City with early, safe, and inexpensive abortions.

Our press releases and public condemnation of the city health community began to hurt. We knew they were hurting when in late October pressure was put on Family Planning Information Service, the official referral agency operated by Planned Parenthood, to stop giving our telephone number to women who were having trouble getting hospital abortions. We were very dependent on FPIS for referrals of women having trouble, and the Interagency

Council which represented city health agencies wanted to get advocacy out of the clergy's hands and put it in FPIS where they could control it. Gradually Gordon Chase, Health Services Administrator, began to find out the "truth" about the performance of his hospitals and took steps to rectify that situation. By December, 1970, the situation began to look much better. Clinics began to flourish, and Women's Services, which Dr. Hale Harvey had begun on July 1, proved its capacity to do volume low-cost first trimester abortions in a medically safe setting with counseling and humane treatment. But a year passed before the Health and Hospitals establishment admitted that Clergy and Lay Advocates were right about the impracticality of doing all first trimester abortions at inpatient hospital facilities.

One of the facts that struck us hard in our new role as watchdogs of "hospital abortion performance" was the capacity of structures and bureaucracy to circumvent laws, so that a change in the law which seems like such a significant victory is only meaningful when the new conflicts are identified and resolved. When legal changes come and reform statutes are installed, they are only words in a legislative code and sometimes mean very little. One has only to remember the seeming triumph of the Voting Rights Act of 1964, which was followed by congressional refusal of appropriations to federal officers in southern counties to enforce violations of the people's rights. The new law was an empty victory when it was not accompanied by the creation of new structures that implemented that law in ways which the legislators intended. Being a lobbyist changing and updating laws is relatively easy, but engaging in the reform that makes new laws meaningful is much harder. When the changes do come, one of the surprises in social reform is that some of your "friends" become your "adversaries." For example, many of the people in the health establishment in New York were with us in favoring liberalization of the law, but those same people became our "enemies" as we tried to innovate a new medical delivery system. Those people who saw our activities as a real threat to the status quo had a deep, vested interest in the health and medical profession. They considered our invasion of their field as definitely "meddling." After all, the hospital facility was the standard unit for the practice of medicine, and the suggestion that *hospitals* were not needed for the elective procedure of abortion in the first trimester came as a threat from "outsiders."

This experience was reinforced for us at Judson because we were engaged on a second front in the battle with hospital professionals. In 1968–1969, we helped create and organize for the streets of the East Village a mobile medical unit to service the health needs of young people who were predisposed to stay away from large hospital facilities either for preventive or curative medical service. The large hospital in whose catchment area the mobile unit was located put every obstacle in our path to prevent this experiment from happening. The contention was that only in a "real" hospital with all its resources and backup facilities was it safe to treat diseases and service health needs. We reminded them of the war where frontline medical units worked out of tents in the mud and muck without white walls or uniforms and with a minimum of medical officialism. We opened anyway, and the unit functioned. People who would never darken the doorway of that nearby hospital came with their needs. This experience was another testimony to the powerful, reactionary resistance that people build into organizational status quos. This tendency is the reason that reforms of legal statutes and administrative codes are many times meaningless gestures so that the role of concerned citizen advocacy is an absolute necessity.

As clergy, our involvement with the issue of abortion during a period when no one else was involved, gave us knowledge and credentials in a field which tends to be preempted by professionals, whose prejudices and preferences had never been questioned by nonprofessionals. We knew, for example, that in most hospital units, the Ob/Gyns run the maternity section of the hospital and if abortions were done in ordinary hospitals, not without a certain ambivalence on the part of those making the assignment, the woman who was terminating her pregnancy would be placed in a room with women delivering babies. The psychological trauma resulting from that situation would be cruel treatment for the abortion patient. Our experiences had sensitized us to the woman's fear, anxieties, physical and emotional concerns, and we had no final stake in anything except the woman and her needs. We wanted to make her experience compassionately humane with as little pain and suffering as possible. In the early months after the law was passed, we were outraged when women getting later terminations, up to twenty-two weeks' gestation, were required by the medical authorities in city hospitals to sign a "fetal death certificate" as the "maternal parent of the deceased." This psychological assault upon women was justified by spokesmen who said the Board of Health must keep statistics. Outrages like this coupled with the judgmental and punitive attitudes among hospital personnel were destructive of whatever dignity and self-assurance women might have had. These factors fortified our continuing insistence that new kinds of medical facilities geared to this particular medical procedure must be created and should be encouraged, not hampered, by health agencies.

Another revelation that came to us when the law changed was the new cast of characters that surfaced to join the number of those providing abortion services. In the "illegal" days when we were fighting for liberalization, our friends were mostly social activists, women's rights' advocates, "single issue" reformers, almost all of them with clear motivations. When the law changed, people who claimed their desire was to see that every woman could have an abortion came out of the woodwork claiming to be "humanitarian." These were the "business Mafia," as we called them. From April when the legislature acted, the calls began to come in from bright young business entrepreneurs who wanted to build abortion clinics. They said they wanted our CCS "know-how," but what they really wanted was our *clients*. At that time some fifty to sixty thousand women a year were going through our counseling network from Maine to Washington. These businessmen, usually collaborating with a psychiatrist or an Ob/Gyn, were out to make a bundle off a brand-new enterprise. After all, look at what the "illegal abortionist" did for himself in the old days. Now it could be done legally! If you want to understand how "sugar plums danced before their eyes," do a little quick arithmetic: if you performed only 500 abortions a week at $300 per abortion, that's approximately $600,000 a month gross or $7 million a year. You could pay fantastic salaries, buy a building, and still have a phenomenal return on your investment. These entrepreneurs were willing for us to design the facility, set up the services, and be consultants (for a fat fee) all in order that those poor women could get the abortion they so richly deserved!

Then there were all those greedy doctors who, as soon as the law changed, called CCS and Planned Parenthood to volunteer the services they realized would be needed. These doctors were going to perform the first trimester abortions right in their offices. They had already ordered their vacuum aspirators and were ready to give up their day off if it meant picking up $3,000 in an afternoon. We knew one doctor who was head of Ob/Gyn at a hospital with stringent rules for an overnight stay and general anesthesia for early abortion cases, but after urging Health Code rules that restricted all abortions to hospital facilities, he offered to do patients in his office for $300 each. Now there was a physician whose left and right hands were perfectly coordinated! We just had to hang up the phone with loathing for all of these brave, helpful doctors. Where were they when we were begging them to abort a twelve-year-old girl who had been raped and was pregnant? Our bitterness at these doctors was exceeded only by our contempt for them. As far as we were concerned, they were a disgrace to their profession.

The third genre of character that came out into the open when the law changed was the now famous "commercial referral agent," the true entrepreneur of a capitalist enterprise, the middleman who has no skills but doesn't need them because he collects for other people's services. In much of our business world this kind of person is a thoroughly necessary evil whose gains are written into the markup of the prices we pay for that which we consume. One area of professional life where there is no middleman is the medical and health field. Even the hint of such, i.e., fee splitting among doctors, is considered a breach of medical ethics. One of the first such agents was a businessman who started operating charter flights to Europe and who ended up under investigation in New York State for violation of the law. It is rumored that he creamed millions of dollars off the top of the abortion business at the expense of women. This latter group of referral agents became the source of attack by the CCS and Planned Parenthood in New York City. Our efforts resulted in a law which made illegal the operation of commercial abortion referral organizations. Although this effort did not stop them entirely, it did put the law on the right side of the issue.

The story of our struggle against commercial referral agencies is worth setting down because it was an unexpected complication that accompanied the liberalization of abortion. The situation was exacerbated by the differentiation of abortion statutes in different states. In one state, a woman may be completely forbidden to have a therapeutic abortion, except when her life is endangered, but in a neighboring state the law may have been reformed or repealed. The "middleman" or a commercial referral agency plays the role of helping the woman get from A to Z, terminate her pregnancy, and get back home. When CCS began its counseling service in 1967 before the laws were changed, one of the tasks was referral, putting a woman in contact with an accredited and competent source of care for terminating her pregnancy. In that sense the clergy acted as a source of information. In the "illegal" days that information was very important, but when the law changed and abortion became simply another elective medical procedure, there was a real question whether there needed to be a person between the woman and the doctor or hospital and clinic.

Soon after the law changed in New York and it could be seen that New York City would be the "abortion capital of the United States," commercial referral services sprang up everywhere. Sometimes they were "front organizations" for a group of doctors running an abortion group practice; other times they were independent agents setting up contracts with abortion clinics and hospitals where the agent was paid so much for every referral. The situation was really no different from when the Mafia offered CCS $50 per woman for abortion referrals to their "doctors" in New Jersey. Most of the doctors and clinics who went into business had no other way of getting patients except stealing them from each other, which they blatantly did at La Guardia airport by having their driver pick up the other clinic's patient. Many an unsuspecting woman got her abortion in a different place than where she had made an appointment.

When the New York CCS ended referral service, we believed that we were doing the right thing so as not to tie the clergy permanently into the procedure. In retrospect we probably made a mistake in disbanding before we could see what would happen with the growth of the commercial agents in New York. Nevertheless, our decision was to move into advocacy and to turn referral over to Family Planning Information Service, which was nonprofit and which would give free information as well as help arrange abortions for women in New York hospitals.

In the winter of 1971 after the commercial services had been exposed for highly exploitative and brazen fee-splitting arrangements with doctors, the office of the attorney general in New York

State opened hearings on the problem. In our first testimony before his committee, we supported the regulation of the commercial services rather than outlawing them because we were worried about overburdening our Clergy Services across the country; we had no desire to make it more difficult for a woman to find a referral source that was reliable, even if she did not use Clergy Services or Planned Parenthood.

But we changed our minds in the next two weeks and gave written testimony to the attorney general's office of that fact. We said that the commercial services should be outlawed, not regulated, because, given the way they functioned, they usurped the prerogatives and responsibilities of the medical profession in regard to the patient/physician relationship; if they were made legal, even with restraints, the practice would set a dangerous precedent for commercial middlemen in all areas of health care. The major argument *against* outlawing them was that women would not be able to get abortions. But that was a spurious argument since the women we were concerned about were out-of-state women and for the most part the white, middle-class people who have always found their way to help. Other women, the marginally poor, ghetto women, were not being helped by these commercial referral services anyway. The poor had to rely on the clergy who could care for a limited number because they referred largely to a nonprofit clinic which willingly accepted as patients a certain number of poor women.

The final resolution of this matter came with the passage of a bill which banned profit-making commercial referral services operating in the state of New York. CCS and Planned Parenthood were allowed to continue making referrals because they did not charge women a fee for information and had no kickback arrangements with any clinic or hospital.

The law struck at the heart of every enterprise making money by charging a fee for information about the source of medical assistance. Section 4501 of Article 45 stated:

No person, firm, partnership, association or corporation, or agent or employee thereof, shall engage in for profit any business or service which in whole or in part includes the referral or recommendation of persons to a physician, hospital, health related facility, or dispensary for any form of medical care or treatment of any ailment or physical condition. The imposition of a fee or charge for any such referral or recommendation shall create a presumption that the business or service is engaged in for profit.

We believe the example set by the experience of hundreds of clergy and lay counselors who gave thousands of hours of uncompensated time resulted in passage of that law which cannot help but abound to the benefit of consumers of medical services.

The narrow and unrelenting stand we had taken requiring that Clergy Services be free of any but voluntary contributions was clearly exonerated by the distinction the New York law made between clergy and other referral services. Once abortion was legal, some persons in our Clergy Services believed it was only fair to charge a fee for counseling women. The question was understandable. After all, the clergy weren't paid for this counseling, and their own expenses for telephones and running their local CCS many times came out of their pockets; so, to defray their own expenses, it was natural for them to consider asking for a surcharge on patients sent to Women's Services. Although the request seemed reasonable, we were adamantly opposed to the clergy charging women or getting what would amount to a "kickback" from the clinic, and the idea was never pursued.

This issue was deep at the heart of what CCS had been about since its origin. We did not believe that any counseling that was a part of the ministry of the church ought to be paid for by the recipient, except voluntarily. This conviction was particularly true in regard to abortion counseling, as in this instance women were forced to go to clergy who had information they needed and couldn't get elsewhere. To place a price on the service smacked of the "sale of indulgences," especially to those outside of the church. The church had made a lot of theological talk over the past decade about servant-people serving the world as well as the church, but when it came right down to practice, the temptation was there to charge some money for counseling those who weren't part of our churches.

One reason that Clergy Services attained the reputation they did around the country, particularly in the days in which abortion was illegal, was that there was a high level of professional counseling and no money passed hands. In all the times that we were making arrangements with "illegal" abortionists, though they were charging unscrupulous prices to women, we never accepted any offers of money. We easily could have rationalized in those days that the doctors should pay for the running of CCS because of the excellent job of screening that our counselors were doing. When we were offered money, which was not all that often, we always suggested to the doctor that he could keep it and apply it against lowering the price of abortions.

A further ethical consideration related to the new law which was passed in New York State against commercial referral agencies was the precedent that information and/or arrangements for medical assistance and services is not a salable commodity. Otherwise, why not such arrangements for all medical services? These entrepreneurs saw in the abortion referral business the possibility of making a fast buck during a transitional period in medical practice. They were charging a woman anywhere from $10 to $100 for information; one of the *real* distinctions between Clergy Services and other referral groups was that the clergy did not charge any fees.

Finally another important consideration in arranging "kickbacks" for referrals from a clinic has to do with the conflict of interest. For example, if CCS had an arrangement to receive money for its operation from a clinic like Women's Services, and a few months later the price went up and the quality went down, would not our freedom to pull out of that facility be curiously hampered by our dependency on the money that made our operation possible? The integrity of our decision would be seriously jeopardized by such a monetary understanding.

Another unexpected problem met us with passage of the reformed abortion law in New York State. The new law made abortions legal up until the twenty-fourth week. Our experience with second trimester (thirteen to twenty-four weeks) abortions had been minimal during the three years of our operation. We sent all late pregnancies, when the women could afford it, to London or Tokyo. Dr. David Sopher in London performed abortions for several years using the laminaria procedure under general anesthesia. This procedure involved the use of instruments to remove the fetus. Then when our law changed, CCS counselors began sending a fair number (about 200 a week) of late terminations to New York City. The only accepted procedure for late termination in this country is known popularly as the saline method. Briefly, the procedure is as follows: A needle is put through the abdomen into the amniotic sac, and several ounces of fluid are removed and replaced with an equal amount of a highly concentrated salt solution. The salt solution kills the fetus and stops the release of placental hormones. The patient within a twenty-four-hour period undergoes labor similar to a live birth, and the fetus and placenta are then expelled with the help of labor-producing medication.

Clearly, most women did not voluntarily wait that long to decide to terminate their pregnancies. However, if a woman was ten or eleven weeks pregnant when she was initially examined, the task of getting to a counselor, receiving information, getting together her resources, and making arrangements to travel some five hundred to a thousand miles distance meant that she would be past the twelve-week period during which abortions could safely be performed in a clinic using vacuum aspiration. This meant then that she must wait until the sixteenth week before she could obtain a saline abortion. The psychological pressure upon the woman who had to carry the fetus another month after her decision was a traumatic one. If you add to that pressure the nature of the later procedure which was more dangerous and difficult, one can understand what happened to women.

We got our first inkling of trouble when the reports from clergy across the country began to indicate some bad psychological and emotional reactions to the late termination. What we discovered was that in this medical procedure the woman literally had to go through a "mini-birth" in which she passed the fetus in bed. Often she saw the fetus and was highly disturbed. A woman who had a miscarriage but was forced during the D & C to look at the products of conception would have a similar reaction. For most women who had the fears and anxieties of having to wait so long, it was an extremely disturbing situation.

It became clear to us that this method of evacuation, the only common procedure used by the medical profession in this country, was highly undesirable and worked an inordinate hardship on women. The contrast between our experience with late terminations in England with Dr. Sopher was so striking that we began to raise questions about why the American medical profession did not use the laminaria method which seemed so much more humane and satisfactory for the patient. We were told by every doctor we asked that laminaria was a very unsafe and even dangerous procedure. These reports were not borne out by the complication rate on late abortions in England or Japan where the laminaria technique is practiced, and we were highly puzzled. However, we were left with no alternative but to suggest that all counselors prepare counselees with late pregnancies for a very taxing and difficult time in order to be sure they understood what lay ahead and would be able to decide on that basis whether to have an abortion or to carry the pregnancy to term. Unfortunately, most of these patients were teenage girls, who had been afraid to tell their parents, or ghetto women who simply didn't know that they were pregnant until very late, and had difficulty locating a source of help.

In order to understand the nature of the operation and its emotional effect upon women, National CCS employed Sonja Hedlund to spend three months as an observer in hospitals where saline abortions were being done. At the end of that time she issued a report on her findings and made recommendations for pre-abortion counseling. Copies of this report were sent to all CCS counselors around the country for use as a guide. We did not find out until almost a year later the real reason why the saline method is the only generally approved late termination technique in this country. A physician using laminaria on an experimental basis in a West Coast hospital spoke to us about the sharp contrast between the two methods. In the saline method, the burden is on the woman to pass the products of conception; so she thereby has to deal with a sixteen- to twenty-four-week fetus, while with laminaria the doctor must remove the fetus with instruments. Such a procedure would probably be almost as traumatic for many doctors as the saline procedure is for women. This explanation seemed more plausible than any other we had heard and confirmed our feelings that doctors develop prejudiced practices and justify them with statistical mendacity that makes the layman believe that a particular procedure is used in order to save life when, more probably than not, it is used to save the doctor time, unpleasantness, or money. In that sense the medical profession is no different from others; lawyers give professional advice that lands clients in jail because it concludes a case more quickly; clergy use theology to justify a course of ethical behavior to a parishioner. One could swallow the phony explanations from doctors more easily if one did not have to endure the high and mighty medical pretensions, couched in jargonese.

Women would be greatly benefited if the medical profession could develop a new procedure that is both safe and humane for late termination of pregnancy. Such an effort would seem only fair if doctors do not have the stomach for dealing with the "products of conception."

The changing of law is simplicity itself compared with the complexity of its implementation. Every state where reformers, clergy and lay alike, are fighting for change needs to have a group whose sole task is to lay the groundwork for what will happen when the law changes. Some states have liberalized abortion laws but women still cannot get abortions because of excessive price, red tape, or simply lack of planning for medical facilities and doctors to perform services. The laws on abortion in Alabama and Kansas, for example, allow extensive freedom for abortion procedures, but the women of those states are still traveling thousands of miles to obtain a medical service which the laws of their own state allow. They have to do so because no group of people planned for what would happen when the law changed. For example, a first trimester abortion in a hospital in Topeka, Kansas, costs $500; so many Kansas women fly to New York City and get an abortion for $125. Even allowing for air fare, the cost is far less than the termination would cost a woman in her own hometown.

The experience of CCS was a hard but valuable teacher for all of us, and the abortion issue provided a testing ground for a great variety of rhetoric and strategies that have grown up around social change. Some of those lessons may be profitable for other fields of social reform.

Lessons We Learned in Social Change

Our particular struggle for social change and legal reform in relation to abortion came at a time when the youth revolution was in full swing, anti-war activity was gaining social and political momentum, and radical politics was breaking out on campuses and in the streets of this country. By comparison our campaign with its long-range "conservative" strategies and pragmatic tactics seemed almost counterrevolutionary and certainly not very significant except to a few people.

In our role of giving leadership nationally we often devised policies and followed practices that seemed unnecessarily cautious, and our critics assailed us and even our colleagues doubted us from time to time. But that cautious campaign was related to goals and purposes that were more important than political "scoring" or ideological victories. To reiterate our major reason for being, it was primarily to provide counselors to enable women to get safe, low-cost abortions with a minimum of mental anguish and emotional trauma. Secondarily, we wanted to change the laws that made our presence as counselors necessary. Socially and politically all the things we did in the Clergy Consultation Service were related to these goals and how we would effect them. In retrospect the lessons we learned in the struggle for abortion rights for women were exceedingly important and perhaps need to be recalled for whatever application they may have for other social issues or areas of social change. It is with a sense of humility that we offer these lessons, for they come from no special wisdom or political skill but from the difficult day-by-day struggle with the problem, firsthand, and the agony of decision making that could have at any time doomed what good we were doing. We realize that these cautionary notes we are offering will fall on deaf ears to those who believe that social change or legal reform comes with "revolutionary rhetoric" or the physical destruction of one's opponents. But if you still believe that tactics and strategy may be more important than scoring political points or scaring the establishment, then these lessons may be simply helpful hints worth heeding in the next social crusade.

When we opened the New York CCS in 1967, we were very conscious of at least three natural adversaries: the Roman Catholic Church, the medical profession, and law enforcement agencies. The natural temptation of every social reformer is to attack his enemies, the perpetrators and defenders of injustice. There is in the psychological makeup of every "crusader" a combination of righteous indignation and unflagging zeal that feeds the need to expose the enemy and put him to rout. This natural desire may interfere in ways that sacrifice the "victims" of injustice in exchange for the punishment of the "enemy."

We found that it was hard to resist this temptation. To do so meant putting the "women-victims" before the "cause" of fighting the enemies of progress.

The Roman Catholic Church, if it decided to repeat its performance of the 1940s with its open attack on Margaret Sanger, the advocate of birth-control methods, would be an adversary of sufficient power and influence to produce pressures for closing us down before we opened up. The Protestant and Jewish clergy were in the vulnerable position of not only advocating and assisting women in an act of mortal sin contrary to Catholic morality, but we were also performing an "illegal" act. Our conviction was that this "sleeping giant" should not be awakened by our cries of social outrage; in fact, we thought that no hostile noises should be made at all. We considered our struggle at that time to be not against the Roman Catholic Church but against an archaic law (put on the books by Protestants) and an apathetic public. We gave the Roman Catholic Church the benefit of a tolerance that it seldom demonstrated. In an article that was a preamble to our action, these words set the tone for our dealing with the Roman Catholic position:

> The time is long overdue for the reform or eradication of the present (abortion) law. . . . It is altogether fitting that the leadership for the reform come from the institution most responsible for its origin and perpetuation, namely, the Christian Church. As for the Catholic Church, it cannot be expected that their theology nor the ethical directions drawn from that

doctrine are going to be negated by the church fathers. However, that doctrine is applicable to Catholics and is not meant to provide any basis for civil law. . . .

As for Protestants who are basically responsible for the beginnings of the law as it now stands, we have a moral and theological imperative to correct this heartless and inequitable law against women. . . .[1]

In the period of time from May, 1967, to the time the law changed in New York State in 1970, the CCS never really received hostile reactions or any public pressures from the Roman Catholic Church against the work we were doing. There was a "live and let live" attitude in our relationship that postponed for several years the all-out warfare between the Roman Catholic Church and others over the abortion issue.

The second natural adversary of clergy involvement with the abortion issue was the medical profession. This is not to say that all doctors were opposed to a change in the law or resented the fact that clergy were counseling women about a medical problem. The fact that abortion was "illegal" except for therapeutic (sic!) reasons gave the gynecological profession the excuse it needed for refusing their patients the help they required. Many doctors who are supposedly the practitioners of medical science and who pride themselves on objectivity suddenly, before this issue, became moralistic and punitive, refusing help in even the most desperate situations. We will never forget the mother whose twelve-year-old daughter had been molested by a baby sitter and had become pregnant. Fighting for the future of her child, she had pounded on every medical door she knew. At the last hospital she visited the gynecologist and the psychiatrist took the child into their office and, in order to avoid any treatment or responsibility, asked her the most "obscene" question I can remember; they said, "Dear, wouldn't you like to be a mummy?" The mother, enraged, took her child and left, finally ending up in our office.

Scenes like this, and they were myriad, gave us every reason to attack the medical profession for its cowardice and abdication in the performance of professional duties. We easily could have opened up on their immoral and inhumane actions regarding their women patients and their willingness to use an "impossible" law to avoid moral culpability and legal risk on behalf of their patients.

---

[1] Howard Moody, "Man's Vengeance on Woman," *Renewal Magazine,* February, 1967, p. 7.

However, those doctors were a group of people we needed. We wanted them to do pelvic examinations and prepare medical notes in order that we might serve women more effectively.

Finally, law enforcement agencies were a third natural adversary. After all, we were involved in a practice that had every possibility of being declared a criminal act. The language of the 1967 statute in New York State was at least ambiguous enough to warrant a judgment that those who openly "aided and abetted" in the procurement of an abortion were guilty of a crime. We easily could have held press conferences and issued releases telling about a group of clergy who were engaged in a dramatic act of civil disobedience, inviting the police or the district attorney to do their duty. Then when they did act, we could have attacked the law enforcement officers for going after poor women and clergy instead of tracking the Mafia and arresting "muggers." The police certainly would have complied; a minister or rabbi would have been arrested; we would have hogged the headlines for a couple of days; and some loud speeches would have been made on the persecution of preachers, but thousands of women (who subsequently went through the CCS) would have gone without help.

One lesson we learned was not to clobber the opposition and label them for what they were. Such an approach would have made us feel good at times but probably would not have served our concerns. Many a reform fight and effort for social change has gone down the drain because it is more dramatic and exciting to fight in public real or mistaken enemies than it is to do drudge work as servants of a cause, in this instance, women and their right to control their reproductive processes.

Another lesson we learned in the abortion rights struggle involved the dangers and difficulties of becoming preoccupied with a single issue, such as abortion. We had to fight continually against being labeled as experts on abortion or being thought of as social activists concerned only with abortion. The occupational disease of every social crusader for a cause is myopia.

We discovered how easy it is to slip into judging all political action or all candidates on the basis of *our* issue. We had to keep reminding ourselves that abortion is one small part of a much larger picture of family planning, population control, and ecological disaster. We met lots of people in the abortion rights movement who seemed to eat, sleep, and breathe abortion problems. These people were so inordinately preoccupied with this single issue that they seemed not to recognize that the world was suffering from any other ills that mattered. Sometimes we wondered what these people would do if there were no longer an "abortion issue," and we felt perhaps they would retire from the human race satisfied that the millenium had come. We never believed for a moment that abortion, for instance, was a more important issue than self-determination for black communities or the rape of Indochina or fighting an unconstitutional draft or working with César Chávez to unionize farm workers. However, we never seemed to lack for reformers, whose label of arrogance is never simply attributed but truly earned, who believe that if you are not engaged in *their* piece of the action that somehow you are a traitor to the revolution.

Anyone would have to have an incredible insolence to accuse a black preacher colleague, up to his eyeballs in confrontations with community militants, of not caring about women because he refuses to take a public stand on abortion. No one has more than a fragment of the truth or a piece of the action—one small handle to turn so that some human suffering is eased, an injustice amended, or some priorities rearranged. Only an enlarged ego or fanatical fantasy can turn that single issue or reform into a major source of the world's salvation.

The time that this single-issue distortion struck the hardest was after the abortion law had changed and we were engaged in a legislative lobbying effort in New York State to defend the liberal law. We spent a number of days in the legislative halls, cornering reticent legislators running for their political lives against "Right-to-Lifers" threats. There were a number of significant bills before the legislature: bussing, desegregated housing, civil liberties issues, and many more. However, we were buttonholing and browbeating every politician only on the subject of abortion as if nothing else he did or thought mattered in that legislative session. Coming back to New York City on the plane, we sang our *"mea culpas"* because we had spent all that time and energy with politicians, even had promised to support some in upcoming campaigns, all in exchange for the *right* vote on the abortion law. We felt a little dirty at the end of the session, not because we were involved in lobbying and political manipulation, but because all of it was done on behalf of a single issue. More than ever the experience caused us to appreciate all those other people engaged in fighting for other causes.

All of us must recognize that circumstances and Providence put some of us in a particular place at a particular time. One time Bill Coffin was in the office at the height of his involvement with the draft and the war in Vietnam. And he said, "Moody, I'm glad you are doing the abortion business. I feel badly that I can't do more myself, but I refer them on to you." And Moody told Bill he was thankful for his witness and work in the anti-war movement and wished he could do more there. We ought to rejoice when our colleagues are engaged in issues other than our own that are also very vital, knowing that there are other dimensions of the human problem. Surely the immensity and complexity of the social issues that face this nation ought to protect any wise activist from the arrogance that believes only one issue is important.

Another lesson that we learned in our attempt at social change and legal reform is that neither theorizing nor theologizing is ever a substitute for immersion and personal involvement in the issue. In the early days of the formation of the CCS in New York City, a minority of the clergy thought that we ought to study the issue for a year before we took any action such as counseling women. The ancient, churchly solution to problems is to study them, appoint a committee, write a report, and file it for future reference. But we refused that well-worn path of cogitation and procrastination and plunged into the problem, comforted by Bonhoeffer's admonition, "You will not know what you will not do."

Most of the clergy had no experience with the act of abortion or of counseling with women whose pregnancy was unwanted. It was a new world, and almost every person's mind was changed by confrontation with the issue in the form of a real, live woman anguishing and anxious about how she could prevent this fateful fact from ruining her life without destroying herself in the process. She could not afford the luxury of a year's study or a few lectures in moral theology. The embryo was growing and she had to decide, and counselors soon learned that each day's delay prolonged the agony and increased the dangers. Our day-to-day work taught us how few women wanted abortions for the reasons most liberals conceded were justifiable. When we started, most of us favored some liberalization of the law, but within a six-month period every clergy (seeing between fifteen and twenty women per week) believed passionately not in liberalization but in repeal of the law. Many people heralded the reform law in Colorado as a milestone, and it probably seemed like that to prestigious professionals, such as members of the American Law Institute who were concerned with legal niceties and the appearance of reforming the law, but who had not had experience with women seeking an abortion.

In the battle for social change or legal reform, ideology (whether textbook or mimeographed) is hardly ever a reliable index to what reform should be made. A number of theologians of the armchair variety chastised the involved Protestant clergy because they were influenced so much by their pastoral responsibilities that they had neglected the weightier matters of theological ethics. The translation of that criticism made by our theological elders meant that we were letting human pain and practical needs of women who were crying out for the right to control their reproductive functions take precedence and priority over all the preordained orders of the dogmatics we had been taught to revere. We Christian ministers, who were the repository of faith to be taught and passed along with a kind unerring consistency, had succumbed to the expediency of dealing with day-to-day realities, sacrificing ethical "principles" for pragmatics of human need. We let women's rights predominate "God's orders"; we gave the freedom of a woman to choose preeminence over the rights of a fetus to be born. We forsook the teaching of our masters, Barth, Brunner, Bonhoeffer, in order to be a pastor to women who needed us.

The history of social movements is full of people who tried reform by the book. Whether the ideology is religious or political, it seldom leaves room for the human quotient which requires compassion and empathy for persons rather than correctness of political and religious doctrine. In the fight for abortion rights for women there was no substitute for daily absorption in women's problems. That involvement taught us that the people who thought about abortion reform lacked the depth of analysis to envision the change that would be required to give women real freedom over their lives in the area of their reproductive functions.

Another lesson we learned in the growth and development of the CCS was *that reform is often the enemy of real change.* When the abortion issue was removed from hushed conversations to public debate, the solutions began to be formulated. By far the most popular and oft-proposed resolution of the issue beginning around 1967 was the American Law Institute's proposed reform measure, which allowed abortion in instances when the pregnancy was caused by rape or incest, when the fetus was malformed, or when there was a serious threat to the health of the mother. Governor Rockefeller in 1967 appointed a distinguished panel to recommend changes in the abortion law in New York. They commended the American Law Institute's abortion reform model law, and our CCS came out against the report. The following is an excerpt from the CCS response to the governor's committee:

The report which is reported to call for "vast liberalization" will be of little help in assisting thousands of women seeking termination of their pregnancy. All the proposed measure will do is to make doctors less hypocritical, and it will only make *legal* what is being done by doctors and hospitals now. The measures proposed have the effect of putting a band-aid on a cancer. The genuine social problem of abortion requires more radical amelioration if it is to be of any real consequence!

Less than one year of experience had taught our counselors that under a so-called "liberalized" abortion law only about 5 percent of the women whom they saw would qualify for an abortion. The political pragmatist warned us that coming out for repeal of the abortion law was politically naïve and practically hopeless. But our work with thousands of women had taught us that anything less than repeal would be liberal window dressing covering a deadly status quo, and the public would be conned by the appearance of change. Many people believed that the liberalized law passed in Colorado in 1967 was a great step forward until the end of the first year when it was announced there was an actual decline in the number of abortions done. Our experience had taught us that 90 percent of the women seeking abortions would not get them under the reform law, and in addition the reform law would be as discriminatory as the old law. The people who had means, access to doctors and private hospitals, or a history of psychiatric treatment would be affected. The poor, the minorities, and the young would not be the beneficiaries of such a law. The only real change would be complete repeal of the law and that seemed too revolutionary at the time. Plenty of people were willing to settle for a little reform thus forfeiting whatever future opportunity there might be for real change. In too many movements for social change we are too quickly satisfied with small reforms, deluding ourselves into believing that we really have changed something when begrudging legislators shift slightly the burden of an oppressive law. Sometimes even experienced activists who like to think of themselves as "political realists" are bought off with an empty promissory note.

A related lesson we learned in the work we did on abortion repeal is that changing the law doesn't cure or correct social ills; it just removes legal encumbrances. The previous chapter was a catalog of what happens once the law is changed. The elation of winning a battle for legal reform is quickly dissipated by the specter of other problems that legalization surfaces. The whole commercial referral business that we fought threatened to defeat the major purpose of low-cost abortions by adding the cost of a middleman to the price women paid for an abortion. In the "illegal days" those entrepreneurs were not around when women truly needed help to get an abortion.

Laws may be changed overnight, but their implementation may expose a host of new problems. For example, when the abortion law was repealed in New York, we faced a whole health delivery system (doctors, nurses, and hospitals) that was unsympathetic and even resisted changes in attitude and practices regarding abortion. "Illegal abortionists" in the old days would never treat a patient with the hostility and punitive attitudes accorded women in New York hospitals right after the law had changed. Laws are easily altered, but mores, taboos, and morals die very slowly. We discovered that even while the glow of a legal victory yet burned, the world of abortions had not changed much. Women wanting abortions still felt guilty and ambivalent; doctors performing them were either very greedy or felt they were violating the purposes of their medical practice; people working on abortion wards felt they were assisting in murder. The psychological and moral proscriptions that have shaped our minds on this matter will change more slowly than the laws making abortion permissible.

How short are our memories in this regard? Somehow even the most sophisticated political activists in America continue to display an enormous amount of faith in the efficacy of legal reform to correct social ills. We thought the Voting Rights Act of 1964 would give Blacks the vote immediately, or the *Brown* v. *Board of Education* would mean integrated quality education.

What eludes this naïve faith in legal reform to bring about social change is recognition of the immense intransigence of human beings and the social systems which they build that avoid any meaningful transformation of the status quo. When a good liberal. abortion law is passed in the state capital, what remains untouched by that reform is a gigantic, conservative, and bureaucratic medical delivery system which is reluctant to shift gears and create a new mechanism that would insure *all* women an early, safe, and low-cost abortion. No wars are won in social change when laws are passed; only an important battle is won. The hard and difficult struggle is in changing minds and reshaping institutions to accommodate new possibilities that lie ahead.

The last lesson is a truism and can be stated in a single sentence: There are no final victories in social reform without continuing vigilance on behalf of the hard-won victories. In regard to the new abortion law in New York State, the most liberal and far-reaching in the nation, there are those who will not admit that this law should stay on the books. The Roman Catholic Church, led by the Archdiocese of New York and a few Protestants and Jews, has been providing large financial resources for reversing the repeal action or crippling its intent with restrictive amendments. In the next chapter we will look at the parameters of that conflict and its implications for religious peace in America.

The Aftermath of Abortion Reform: The Seeds of Religious Warfare

We are experiencing at this present time in our American life probably the most serious threat to our religious peace and pluralistic coexistence in the past one hundred years. Only the most ignorant or the most callous persons can be oblivious to what can be only a portentous prelude to open religious warfare in our communities and the disruption of the amicable existence of very diverse religious groups in our society. During the last two decades we have witnessed important steps to understanding and toleration among all the major religious groups in the nation. Christians acknowledged, confessed, and began to correct the deep sources of anti-Semitism inherent in their faith. Under the influence of Vatican II, the Roman Catholic Church began to modify and rectify some of their harsh anti-Protestant views; Protestants under the tutelage of persons like Reinhold Niebuhr, John Bennett, and John Courtney Murray began to temper the bigotry born of their Reformation heritage and American nativism. The ecumenical movement, though high level and theological, promised at least a more tolerant and sensitive living together in the American proposition.

But something new in the conflict of values has begun to surface again, almost imperceptibly, in the Roman Catholic Church's effort to save the parochial school system and the ancient, prohibitory abortion statutes. In New York State as well as other places, the escalation of the religious struggle in its more recent manifestations became apparent in the debate over aid to parochial schools. In the fight over the Blaine Amendment in 1967 to allow such aid, there was a low-keyed, but devious Madison Avenue advertising campaign which insinuated invidious charges against anyone who might on principle oppose direct aid to parochial education. Open warfare emerged in the shrill, no-holds-barred battle to kill the present New York abortion law, one of the most liberal in the U.S.

In order to understand the conflict of values and theology that is becoming apparent in the controversy over abortion, we must comprehend a truth about our common life in America that is often denied or ignored: the civil amity and the religious harmony we are able to display from time to time present a fragile surface of unity, but underneath there is passion, and wars are going on. Neither phony brotherhood weeks, nor occasional bursts of ecumenical euphony, nor even the common ties of national chauvinism can serve to hide the deep differences and fervent disagreements of our religious beliefs and morality. Our memories need be jogged only slightly to recall the bitter religious rivalry of other times and places and those silent gaps of misunderstanding that so often characterized Catholic-Protestant and Jewish-Christian relationships in the past. Who doesn't remember those vicious and intolerable stereotypes of each other that we carried, the bad recollections of our former hatreds? After all, the dissonant noise of school boards bickering over religious symbols in the classroom seemed harmless indeed compared with Roman Catholic homes being burned to the ground and pitched battles in the streets of Philadelphia only a hundred years ago. Only a dozen years ago it was alleged that John F. Kennedy should not be president of the United States because he would be loyal first to the pope and the Roman Catholic Church and only secondarily loyal to his country. Many people voted against him because they shared that belief. No one who makes fun of our "new harmony" could wish for the theological fratricide of our past.

Those who wish for true peace based upon social reality must accept two unavoidable premises about the nature of our American experience: (1) There are *real* beliefs and moral values that divide us so that our differences must not be buried in false unity and superficial harmony. (2) Since those differences exist and the structures of "passion" and "war" are just beneath the surface, the concept of "limited warfare" between differing faiths and ideologies offers the best possibility for contributing to justice in the balancing of interests and claims of diverse religious groups. If all religious groups in our democracy would accept the principle of "limited warfare," we could plan for the conflicts that are bound to occur when divergent faiths present their demands in an open and heterogeneous society. In "limited warfare" the aim is never annihilation or unconditional surrender of the opposition. The weapons of "limited warfare" are argument and rational debate with compromise, accommodation, and a reasoned respect for the others' point of view. The health and vitality of our religious communities in America may well be determined by the way in which we do battle in the common social and political order.

In the light of these foregoing principles we must view with alarm the growing escalation of religious warfare evidenced in the latest activities of the leaders of the Roman Catholic Church (from cardinal to priest), the National Right to Life Committee, and even the president of the U.S.A. The first offers the theological rationale and moral absolutes; the Right to Lifers contribute the demonstration and action that follow when a layman's inordinate zeal is untempered by the prelates' pragmatic and cloistered hortatory; and the last adds the imprimatur of the highest office of the land. We need to look at the nature of all of these adversaries of a woman's free choice to terminate an unwanted pregnancy and observe who they are, what they represent, and what fundamental moral and political issues they are raising by their attacks.

First, we should deal with the hierarchy of the Roman Catholic Church, including the office of the cardinal in New York State, the Council of Bishops, and similar church officials. They have, although representing a minority of Catholic believers, denied the principle of "limited warfare" and have through pastoral letter, sermons, and public statements destroyed the spirit of dialogue and debate, opting for sloganeering and religious demagoguery unbefitting our more recent experience in understanding and tolerance. A pastoral letter from thirty Roman Catholic bishops made a verbal assault upon some of our finest and most humane physicians saying, "Abortionists lost no time plying their death-dealing trade. Each day they grow wealthier from the killing of unborn children."[1] In other words, doctors who believe with conviction that it is a woman's right to terminate her un-

---

[1] *New York Times,* December 6, 1970.

desired pregnancy were accused of killing primarily for money. And all persons connected with attempts to effect abortion reform, regardless of the religious conviction and moral values which motivated them to seek more liberal laws, were accused of seeking to establish a policy that would lead to legalized murder.

Now what is new in this stage of our warfare is not the Roman Catholic Church's official position on abortion. This stance has been well-known for some time, as has its public position on birth control, censorship, and other moral issues upon which honest persons, with the same and differing religious persuasions, disagree. What is new is the extremism of the Roman Catholic Church's verbal attacks which smacks of the desperation of "all-out warfare" that will smother the spirit of toleration in bitter divisiveness and return us to an age of religious intolerance and bigotry. Now at issue here is not the right of the Roman Catholic hierarchy to espouse its religious principles and doctrines; that guaranty is written deep in the American political system. What is at issue here, and perhaps more important than where we stand on abortion or aid to parochial schools, is a principle as old as this nation's history, involving how we live together with deep and diverse religious beliefs and ethical viewpoints in a pluralistic society.

The freedom *of* religion is a precious part of our American political experiment. I would presume that all religious groups would applaud the decision of the Supreme Court that the Amish people, a small religious minority, should not be forced against their religious conscience to send their children to public schools. All of the legal accommodations and political forbearance shown toward religious groups in order to assure their freedom of belief and practice are acts which all persons in our democracy must cherish regardless of their religious preference.

In regard to the issue of abortion that is part of our present concern, the state has *no* right to tell the Roman Catholic bishops or the cardinal that they cannot expound their doctrine, expunge their heretical priests, or excommunicate Catholic women for the committing of mortal sin. The government has no right to interfere with the freedom of any religion to function with its theology, dogma, and morality. However, the state has every obligation to refuse to prosecute or criminalize women under legal statutes for an action that one religious group, or at least a portion of its adherents, declares to be a mortal sin subject to ecclesiastical punishment. Such legal action would be a violation of a fundamental principle implicit in the First Amendment to the Constitution, namely, the freedom *from* religion. The Roman Catholic Church leaders have no right to expect the state or its legal system to make punishable the violators of its theological dogmas, its moral canons, or liturgical practices. This principle was involved recently in the case of the "St. Patrick Seven," a group of nuns who protested the war by lying silently prostrate on the floor of St. Patrick's Cathedral. Prostration in Catholic history used to be a bodily act of humiliating penance; now it is grounds for arrest—shades of modernism! The defense lawyer for the nuns based her case on the principle that the state of New York had no right to decide what was a violation of liturgical decorum. When the Roman Catholic Church refused to enter the case, the state dropped the proceedings. We felt that the Archdiocese hoped the nuns would be punished by secular authorities without giving the Roman Catholic Church bad press.

This freedom *from* religion is part of the tradition of our American constitutional system. It is just as clear that the courts of the land should not prosecute Jews who violate Kosher dietary laws or Protestants who carry on sexual practices prohibited by their particular sect or atheists who refuse to take the pledge which says "one nation under God." The principle of the separation of church and state is not an empty axiom but an essential extension of the basic tenet of the freedom *of* and the freedom *from* religion in our American pluralism.

The leaders of the Roman Catholic Church in their use of the language of extremism have reverted to an earlier defensive posture which equated theological and moral differences with "blasphemy" and "treason against God and man." In our differences as religious believers and Americans, we who differ with the hierarchy of the Roman Catholic Church, both Catholic and non-Catholic, have been slandered with names like "murderers." In language and posture the Roman Catholic Church is sowing the seeds of bitter discord. After all, if people are to be called murderers or criminals or unfit to be part of the church, then it's a small step to denying them freedom and locking them up. If in your opinion and according to your belief a person is in error, you may disagree with him, or even feel sorry for him. But if you conclude that person is a "murderer of babies," then you are certain that he or she should be *punished!* We must remind ourselves of the terrible omission deep at the heart of our individual faith. The concept of the rights of, conscience has been since Nuremberg eloquently stated in the Declaration of Human Rights, the Documents of Vatican II, and our own Supreme Court decisions on dissent on the draft and the war. But the seeds of that belief are found in the works of Thomas Aquinas and great cardinals like John Henry Newman. Have the leaders of the Roman Catholic Church forgotten Cardinal Newman's eloquent statement in answer to Gladstone's accusation that Roman Catholics could not be loyal citizens of England owing to their absolute loyalty to the pope? Newman said:

> When God became Creator, He implemented his ethical law, which is Himself, in the intelligence of all his rational creatures. The divine law is the rule of ethical truth—the standard of right and wrong, a sovereign, irreversible, absolute, authority . . . is called conscience and though it may suffer refraction into the intellectual medium of each person . . . still has, as such, the prerogative of commanding obedience.[2]

Or as one of the documents of Vatican II puts it: according to the way a man obeys his conscience, he will be judged. This is not to say that conscience never errs, but even when it is in error, it does not lose its dignity.[3]

In woman's age-long struggle for first-class citizenship and genuine equality in the personhood of the human race, one of the last and most formidable barriers for her is in this area of reproductive rights—the personal and private freedom to determine when and how her reproductive organs will function. That fundamental right is now in most of the states abridged by restrictive abortion statutes. Those women, many of them Catholic and Protestant and Jewish, who have decided under the guidance of their consciences and religious convictions to terminate pregnancies, have been declared "murderers" by those who have for-

[2] John Henry Newman, A Letter Addressed to His Grace the Duke of Norfolk on the Occasion of Mr. Gladstone's Recent Expostulation (1875), pp. 53ff.

[3] "Pastoral Constitution on the Church in the Modern World," in *The Documents of Vatican II*, ed. Walter M. Abbott, S.J. (New York: Association Press, 1966), pp. 213-214.

gotten a fundamental article of faith, the freedom of the individual conscience before God. If by threats and punitive action, conscience is bound and gagged, then all of Christendom is the poorer for it.

In its fight to retain restrictive abortion legislation or to turn back those instances where laws have been liberalized, the hierarchy of the Roman Catholic Church seeks to employ a principle that sets a dangerous precedent at least in our American system where church and state are defined as separate. The Roman Catholic Church is seeking to use the law as the primary sanction to uphold the belief that "abortion is murder." As an article of faith *within* the Roman Catholic Church this belief is not even universally accepted, but within the broader scope of people in this country it certainly is not shared. In a pluralistic culture, to rely primarily on law as a means of attaining conformity of belief is a dangerous precedent. What happens in a nation where beliefs and morality are not homogeneous is described aptly by one of the great moral theologians of the Catholic Church, Father John Courtney Murray, who said:

> Law is indeed a coercive force; it compels obedience by the fear of penalty. However, a human society is inhumanly ruled when it is ruled only, or mostly, by fear. Good laws are obeyed by the generality because they are good laws; they merit and receive the consent of the community, as valid legal expressions of the community's own convictions as to what is just or unjust, good or evil. In the absence of this consent law either withers away or becomes tyrannical.[4]

That statement describes what happens with laws restricting abortion. There is no consent or agreement concerning the law so that when there was only restrictive law, thousands of women all over this country got "illegal" abortions. Since the law has changed in some places, women travel hundreds of miles, pay premium prices, and risk their health at times, because there is no consent to the restrictive law. The law is not enforced; women are not tried and prosecuted for their "crimes." Whether we believe abortion is moral or immoral, right or wrong, it is one of those areas of our moral disagreement that when covered by an unenforceable code creates sham, hypocrisy, and disrespect for law. Once again Father Murray's words are terribly relevant:

[4] John Courtney Murray, S.J., *We Hold These Truths: Catholic Reflections on the American Proposition* (New York: Sheed & Ward, Inc., 1960), p. 167.

The moral aspirations of law are minimal. Law seeks to establish and maintain only that minimum of actualized morality that is necessary for the healthy functioning of the social order. It does not look to what is morally desirable, or attempt to remove every moral taint from the atmosphere of society. . . .

Therefore the law, mindful of its nature, is required to be tolerant of many evils that morality condemns.[5]

Certain practical consequences follow from this understanding of law and morals. If the Roman Catholic Church believes that divorce is absolutely wrong and a violation of God's commandment, the Roman Catholic Church has every right to teach that doctrine and even try to convince fellow citizens of its truth, but it is not right for that church to insist that laws of civil society either prevent or make it extremely difficult for a person to obtain a divorce. If the Roman Catholic bishops and priests want to teach and encourage their followers to refrain from all "artificial" contraceptives in their sexual lives on penalty of committing mortal sin, that is the church's moral business. But to try to enforce legislation or administrative codes that would deny the *choice* of birth-control measures to all people in the society is an excessive use of coercion to compel compliance by all people. If the leadership of the Roman Catholic Church believes that the ovum, the embryo, and the fetus are living human beings, then it only follows that for those who hold that view abortion is never allowable. But on the basis of that doctrine, the Roman Catholic Church should not attempt by legal sanction to deny all women *the choice* of bearing or not bearing an unwanted child.

The action of the hierarchy of the Roman Catholic Church in the excessiveness of its language on the issue of abortion and its all-out warfare to win the *abortion issue* is forsaking some basic tenets of our living together in an open society. Now the issue that suddenly needs open dialogue and serious debate is *not* "when does life begin in the womb?" but "when does freedom of choice and conscience end in society?" The question is not whether "feticide is homicide," but whether in this society any group may impose moral and religious beliefs by legal sanctions upon *all* of society. Analogous to the abortion issue would be the passing of a law that forces a woman, against her religious

5 *Ibid.,* p. 166.

convictions, to terminate a pregnancy or to be sterilized. That law would also be a violation of the belief in the freedom *of* religious practices even when those practices go against the seeming best interest of the state or, in another's view, seem erroneous. The principle of religious liberty to follow the dictates of one's own conscience on matters of faith and morals can never be forsaken regardless of the zeal or conviction with which one holds another's conscience to be wrong. It is of supreme importance as we tackle the complex problems of our social and moral existence together in this nation that we limit the "warfare" by a resolution to refrain from the language of extremism that writes off our opponents as evil adversaries, unworthy of being heard. The leaders of the Roman Catholic Church might seek the humility of our Master to love even the enemy of its own cherished traditions.

If the leadership of the Roman Catholic Church represented the verbal and theoretical base for the coming religious warfare, the Right to Life committees represent the ground troops and commandos of the warfare on the abortion issue. Now the facts ought to be made clear about this vociferous and vocal minority who have surfaced in remarkable fashion in the past five years. There have been certain myths about this vocal minority group that ought to be dispelled. First, it is not a heterogeneous, interracial, interfaith coalition of people. This group represents, for the most part, a certain minority group of lay persons in the Roman Catholic Church. Despite all the efforts to symbolize the mixture of this group, its membership is about 85 to 90 percent Roman Catholic with a few exceptions of well-publicized participants from orthodox Judaism and conservative Protestantism. Another myth about this group is that it is a conspiracy of the Roman Catholic Church, paid for and completely subsidized by that church. There are no facts to substantiate this charge with the exception perhaps of provision of space in which a Right to Life group meets and some militant priests who lend an institutional aura to their makeup. Although the Right to Life group is not conspiratorial in any sense, it is a fanatical minority in the Roman Catholic Church and community and is dangerous, not because it is subversive, but because it is divisive in the deepest sense and as such is a threat to civil peace.

When we label the Right to Life group as fanatics, we are not attempting to lay that charge against individual participants, but we are describing some important characteristics of the group as a whole. One dictionary describes a fanatic as one who has an intense, uncritical devotion. When a person has such a devotion, he tends to believe that all people should believe as he does. So he tries to enforce that belief upon all, denying to others the freedom to act upon the basis of their own belief and conscience. We can see the dangers of fanaticism in the Right to Life stance in terms of its adherents' unquestioned assumptions about abortion and their efforts to enforce their belief upon all others.

The fanatic cannot accept the possibility that the truth which he holds may be partial or limited. When this view of truth is related to ethics, the fanatic's belief that there is no possibility of his being wrong turns an ethical choice into unbearable moral arrogance. However, the fanatic believes so strongly that his truth is indisputable that his actions are, to him, unquestionable.

In the abortion issue, the Right to Life group is fanatical in that they see *no* moral complexity or question involved in the decision to have an abortion. For them, abortion *is* murder. Their visual material uses photographs of a twenty- to twenty-four-week aborted fetus; but according to their theology, at whatever stage the conceptus is terminated—whether an ovum in the second week, an embryo in the third week, or a fetus in the fifth week—the act of termination is a murder, just as if one took the life of a thirty-year-old person.

This view of the biological process gives it a right that transcends any human consideration or intentionality. The biological process is ordained as an Ultimate Good with absolute rights, whether at the stage of ovum, embryo, or fetus. The Right to Life adherent transposes the ovum, embryo, or fetus, by an act of faith, into the repository of spiritual soul and human quality identical to that held by a fully developed human being. The enlarged photograph of the fetus doesn't prove to the Right to Lifer that the fetus is a child—the pictures are simply proof to him of what he already believes. The enlarged photographs are used then to convince the "unbelievers" that in the womb is a fully developed human being. No one can fault this transposition by the fanatic—there is nothing wrong with his act of faith and the ethics he derives from it. But if one is able to infuse the ovum, embryo, or fetus with humanity and spirit (some people do that with animals and insects, and others called "animists" do it with rocks and trees), then it is an easy next step to talk about women and doctors who terminate pregnancies as "murderers."

However, there is an interesting inconsistency in the inordinate concern of the Right to Lifers about abortion and the natural process. About one-third of all the pregnancies in the world are aborted, not by doctors or women or midwives, but by an Unseen Hand called by some religious persons "the will of God" or "natural necessity" (which is translated into natural law). All of these millions of abortions are acceptable because "nature" or "God" dictated that these pregnancies should be aborted for some reason of imperfection or malformation. However, should nature slip up and a physician discover a malformed fetus, neither he nor any mortal for any reason has the right to intercede because "God's will" or "natural necessity" elects that the fetus should be born. If this were not the case, the fetus would have been aborted. Now if there were some consistent concern for the right to life apart from theological assumptions, the devotees would have to protest these absurd and unreasonable abortions—fetuses killed without any good human reasons.

The Right to Life adherent does not seem to find it possible to accept the possibility that he has seen the truth in a distorted and limited way. By converting the embryos and fetuses into an Ultimate Good, he engages in a myopic, "one-dimensional" morality in which the talk of a woman's right is meaningless compared to that of a *deified conceptus*. For him there are no reasons, however persuasive, that could possibly justify not homicide (because we have laws for justifiable homicide) but *deicide*. The deification of the *conceptus* must be as repugnant a form of idolatry to the Holy One as the pagan idolatry which demanded human sacrifice. But the most popular idolatry in which we humans engage is to take finite, partial, and limited truth and by this alchemy of a kind of moral insolence convert it into an absolute value or idol. The mark of the fanatic is nearly always some form of idolatry.

Because fanatics believe that the truth they espouse is not capable of containing any error, they consider compromise and accommodation to be betrayal and their opponent to be not simply wrong but diabolical or evil. Therefore the fanatic is not interested in conversation and dialogue. He seeks only conversion, and his weapons are always slogans and name calling. Of course, if one possesses the only truth and that truth is absolute, it stands to reason that one might be preoccupied with making converts. This form of religious imperialism is not confined to Right to Life adherents. But when people believe that they are the real protectors of life itself, then that belief imparts the kind of zeal which enables them to stand in front of abortion facilities and scream "murder" at women who are following their own beliefs and consciences. Most of us have not been able to condone those who have labeled as murderers members of the armed forces leaving for Southeast Asia to burn and commit mayhem on a whole populace. We respect the conscience that takes one man to war and another to prison in protest against that war. Yet those in the Right to Life groups, most of whom are Catholics in belief and practice, call their coreligionists and sisters "murderers" simply for choosing an elective medical procedure which is allowed by law in certain states. This reaction is a form of cruel and inhuman treatment that only an extreme fanaticism could condone. When children from parochial schools are dismissed and sent to run through the legislative halls with "Abortion Is Murder" labels pasted on their lunchboxes and when legislators are threatened with political extinction if they dare to disagree with the "truth" as it has been revealed, then dialogue has ceased and demagoguery has won.

The Right to Lifers without any exception believe in a compulsory childbearing law (a kind of "forced labor" for all women), which is perhaps one of the last and most formidable blocks against a woman's true freedom and equality. As long as she must forever bear and care for the products of conception, and her mind, body, and spirit are bound by a "biological determinism," she cannot know true liberty. The Right to Lifers might recall a famous American patriot who said, "Give me liberty or give me death." Patrick Henry was not denigrating life or saying it wasn't precious, but he was saying that under certain tyrannies death is preferable. It is a matter of record that some women consigned and required by the law of the land to bear children against their will (which is a kind of legalized rape) have in the past preferred death or the risk of death to living under such oppressive laws. The women in the nation must in due time see the dangers of a compulsory child-bearing law that restricts their freedom of choice and right of conscience whether they be Catholic, Protestant, Jew, or of no religious preference.

Another argument that Right to Lifers have concocted is that there is no such thing as an *unwanted child*. That assertion is used to answer those "bleeding hearts" who keep asking about the fruits of compulsory childbearing laws—unwanted children. This piece of fiction is like saying there are no unwanted blacks in white neighborhoods, no such things as unwanted Jews in WASP enclaves, no unwanted Puerto Ricans in white ethnic strongholds. There are plenty of unwanted children, in orphanages and even in their own homes, and only the most desperate hope could create this gigantic illusion that there are none. Even if wishing could make it so, what about a law that compels women to be "baby-makers" for other women, forcing women to be bearers of the burdens of another's desires? The only thing missing is *free choice*. For the women who love to have babies and give them away it would be wonderful, but for all others an unthinkable bondage.

Finally, a word about the political role in the abortion controversy is in order. Richard M. Nixon lent all the prestige of the office of President of the U.S.A. to help defeat the present liberal law in New York State, which his opponent for the presidency was trying to leave to the decision of the state. Mr. Nixon promoted the question to a national issue by his intervention. It is not extraordinary that Mr. Nixon's view on the worth of human life should be inconsistent or even contradictory, and no one can fault his expressing his own belief on any subject. What is shocking is that he saw fit in his high office to join the hierarchy of the Roman Catholic Church in a public endorsement of its effort to reinstate in New York a compulsory childbearing law that would force every pregnant woman to bear her child, even if it was against her own religious conscience and convictions. That act alone was the most defiant violation of the principle of the separation of church and state in recent history. The intervention of the president of this country in such a highly volatile, religious controversy while it was being deliberated by a state legislature and pending before the Supreme Court can only be interpreted as an action of the most partisan, political opportunism. In a letter to

Terrence Cardinal Cooke commending his efforts to repeal New York's abortion law, the President wrote:

> . . . unrestricted abortion policies . . . seem to me impossible to reconcile with either our religious tradition or our Western heritage. One of the foundation stones of our society and civilization is the profound belief that human life, all human life, is a precious commodity. . . .[6]

Against that one can recall that Richard Nixon has ordered the dropping of more than seven million tons of bombs on Vietnam, killing hundreds of thousands of human beings.

No one can say what the future holds for this issue and the controversy that is abroad in the land, but at this point the Roman Catholic Church has cast caution to the wind in an attempt to retain restrictive abortion laws where they exist and to repeal liberalized abortion laws. For the Roman Catholic leaders this effort is a reckless race against time. The Gallup poll does show an amazing shift in attitudes. In 1968 less than 15 percent believed in liberalized abortion laws. However, in that same year out of a sampling of 6500 women going through our abortion counseling service in New York City, 33 percent were Roman Catholic women. In 1972, 64 percent of persons believed in more liberal abortion laws, and even among Catholics, 56 percent favored liberal laws,[7] in a church where denial of sacraments and excommunication are what one may expect for following one's conscience. This poll bodes well for the future. This trend does not mean necessarily that more Catholic women will get abortions and forsake their church's teaching. It does mean that increasing numbers of all people in this nation, including Catholics, believe that the matter of abortion is something that the law should not dictate, but that every woman must possess the freedom, guaranteed by the Constitution, to follow her religious conscience in the determination of whether she will or will not bear a child.

[6] *New York Times,* May 7, 1972.
[7] *New York Times,* August 25, 1972.

Epilogue

In May, 1972, the model abortion law of New York State, which granted all women freedom of choice in the matter of bearing children, was repealed by the state legislature even though the bill had been highly praised by the President's Commission on Population Growth and the American Future. In its place the legislators passed the Donovan-Crawford bill which permitted abortions only to save the life of the mother. The liberal 1970 law hung on the stroke of a pen, for only Governor Nelson Rockefeller could save it by exercising his veto. The pressure and abuse he was subjected to were phenomenal. In the end he stayed by his convictions which ran contrary to some political realities, and for another year the liberal abortion statute in New York was safe.

In November, 1972, a referendum to liberalize the Michigan abortion law was defeated, despite polls taken two weeks before the vote which indicated that it would be approved by a comfortable majority (60 percent) of the people of that state. When the ballots were counted, 60 percent of the voters had said "No" to change in the existing law. In the political postmortem that followed, the reformers admitted that the last minute all-out campaign by Right to Life forces (into which a reputed million dollars had been poured) was responsible for their unexpected defeat. Billboards and pamphlets portraying the abortion reformers as "murderers" had flooded the state during those last two weeks and the limited assets of those who advocated changing the abortion law were too meager for an effective public reaction.

Those same forces which repealed (but for the grace of Governor Rockefeller) New York's law in May and defeated Michigan's referendum in November are shaping up for another all-out fight in the 1973 session of the New York State Legislature.

If that law falls, thousands of women will be deprived of a

121

fundamental right regarding the freedom to control their own lives and will be forced to live as bond servants to an archaic and vengeful law that at best will be hypocritical and discriminatory. Because other state legislatures may be influenced by the process in New York, the New York State Assembly holds in its hands the fate of millions of women and the progress they have made toward greater freedom and equality. If from fear or by intimidation or political opportunism they vote our mothers, wives, sisters, and daughters into the shame and humiliation of "illegal abortions," they will deserve on their heads the blood of every woman who suffers and dies as a result of their action. For the repeal of the law will not be voted out of ignorance or innocence but with knowledge and forethought because women have already lived in that kind of world and tasted the dregs of punishment for having an unwanted pregnancy.

No more dramatic climax to the long struggle for a woman's freedom of choice could have been envisioned than the announcement of Monday morning, January 22, 1973, that the Supreme Court of the United States had declared it unconstitutional for any state to prohibit abortion during the first six months of pregnancy. This ruling guarantees women the right to choose when and whether they will bear children. It is the vindication of the movement and the work of the clergy begun five and one-half years ago with the conviction that the prohibitory abortion laws were a violation by the state of the woman's right to privacy and personal liberty.